I want
Cosmetic
Surgery,
Now What?!™

by Jodie Green

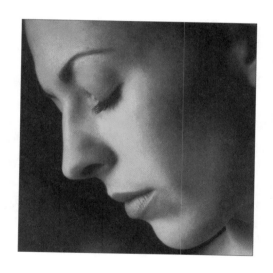

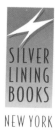

SILVER LINING BOOKS

NEW YORK

For information, contact:
Silver Lining Books
122 Fifth Avenue
New York, NY 10011
212-633-4000

Other titles in the Now What?!™ series:
I'm turning on my PC, Now What?!
I'm turning on my iMac, Now What?!
I'm in the Wine Store, Now What?!
I'm in the Kitchen, Now What?!
I need to get in Shape, Now What?!
I need a Job, Now What?!
I haven't saved a Dime, Now What?!
I'm on the Internet, Now What?!
I just bought a Digital Camera, Now What?!
I'm Retiring, Now What?!
I'm getting Married, Now What?!
I've got a Grill, Now What?!
I need to give a Presentation, Now What?!
I think I need a Lawyer, Now What?!

Titles in the Now What?!™ mini series:
I just got a Handheld Organizer, Now What?!
I just got a Cell Phone, Now What?!

introduction

For several years now Carole has complained that the face she sees in the mirror is somehow older than the person she is inside. "I know aging is natural, but if I don't feel my age, why should I look it?"

Why indeed? Enter **I want Cosmetic Surgery, Now What?!** It's the perfect introduction to the many procedures available today —from ultra simple to fairly complex—that are designed to help you look better. In these beautifully illustrated pages you'll learn how these procedures are done, how long the effects last, what the risks are, and the price range for each. Want to erase wrinkles around your eyes? Consider Botox injections or laser resurfacing (see pages 34 and 54). Concerned about thinning hair? Hair transplants can make a huge difference in your appearance (see page 74). Upset by flabby arms that no amount of exercise can tighten? Liposuction may do the trick (see page 140). And if you want to improve your smile, there's a whole chapter on cosmetic dentistry.

Chic doesn't just happen—it takes research and a good plastic surgeon. The information is in these pages, including how to find and interview the right doctor and dentist. So read on and see if a new you beckons.

Barb Chintz
Editorial Director, the *Now What?!*™ series

table of contents

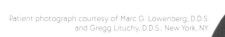

Patient photograph courtesy of Marc G. Lowenberg, D.D.S.
and Gregg Lituchy, D.D.S., New York, NY

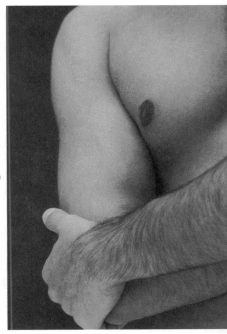

Chapter 1

A New You

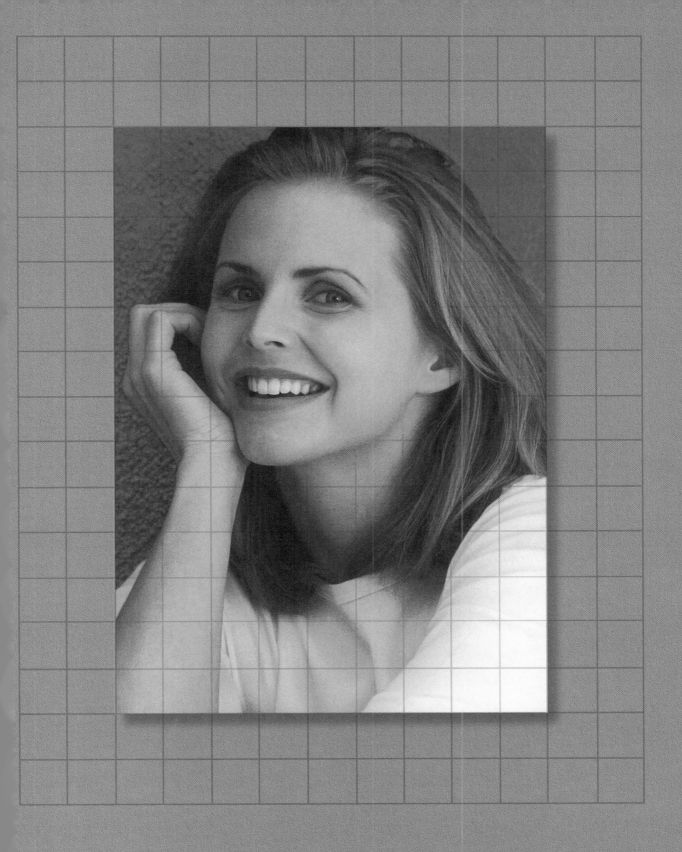

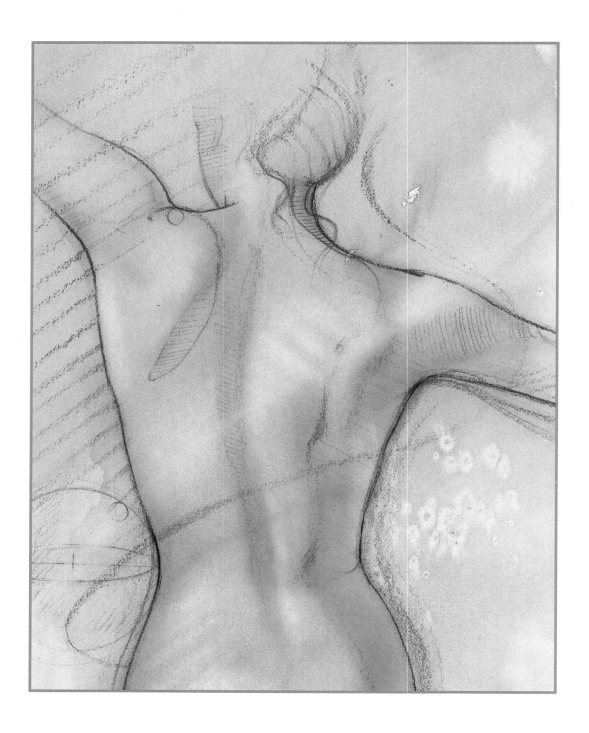

Wanting to look your best is not a symptom of vanity or me-generation narcissism. In fact, it's a sign of sound mental health. That's because a positive self-image is often the backbone to strong self-esteem. The goal of cosmetic surgery is not to make us look better to others, it's to make us look better for ourselves.

what is cosmetic surgery?

And what can it do for you

Maybe, like millions of others, you've been unhappy with the bump on your nose, the shape of your chin, or your receding hairline. Perhaps you've been toying with the idea of increasing your bust or decreasing your thighs. Or, despite your best efforts, you've begun to lose the battle against time and now look older than you feel. Enter cosmetic surgery, which is a form of plastic surgery that reshapes healthy, normal parts of the face or body. The goal of cosmetic surgery is **aesthetic**—to enhance appearance. Don't confuse it with **reconstructive** surgery, which repairs abnormalities caused by birth defects, disease, or trauma.

But there's a lot more to cosmetic surgery than meets the eye. Cosmetic surgeons have long noted that even minor cosmetic changes can do wonders for a person's self-esteem. The other good news about cosmetic surgery is that, thanks to medical advances, many of the procedures can be done on an outpatient basis, with little time off for recovery. Yes, of course there are risks but, thanks to new and better techniques, those too are being reduced. Even so, enter into cosmetic surgery thoughtfully—you want to choose the smallest procedure that will yield the largest benefit for the least risk and inconvenience. Whether you are ready to take the plunge or are just curious about what a new you would look like, read on and find out.

ask the experts

What are the most popular cosmetic surgery procedures?

According to the American Society of Plastic Surgeons, the top five procedures are nose reshaping, liposuction, eyelid surgery, breast enlargement, and the facelift. (All these procedures are discussed in the following chapters.)

Won't cosmetic surgery make me look suddenly different?

Good cosmetic surgery should not be perceptible to others as such—the result should look natural and be consistent with your own unique physical characteristics. You want to find a surgeon who is adept at improving individual features so they fit harmoniously with your face and body. The goal is to have people compliment you on looking healthy and fit.

Is there a difference between a cosmetic surgeon and a plastic surgeon?

The titles are not synonymous. Any physician can call himself a cosmetic surgeon, which is an unregulated term. Plastic surgeons are certified to do both cosmetic and reconstructive work (see more on this on page 15), and typically undergo the most extensive training. This does not mean that a doctor who calls himself a cosmetic surgeon is not skilled at what he does—quite the opposite may be true—but it does mean that if you are considering one you need to ask the right questions about board certification, training and experience, and professional affiliations (see page 190).

your expectations
What's really motivating you

While cosmetic surgery can bring about transformations in people, it is not the surgery itself that is doing the transforming, it's the boost to the person's self-esteem that is enacting the real change. Cosmetic surgery can't get you a promotion if you aren't qualified or save a faltering marriage, but it can give you a new sense of confidence that might make a difference in your life.

Because your expectations are so important, you need to ground them in reality before you undergo any cosmetic procedure. The person seeking to improve a particular problem with his or her appearance will have a much better outcome than someone who is looking for a total makeover.

Search your heart and see what exactly is motivating you to consider cosmetic surgery. There are psychological expectations (Will I feel better about myself? Can I restore my lost youth?); surgical expectations (How much will it hurt? How bruised and battered will I look right after the operation?); and social expectations (Will people notice a change and treat me differently?). Those who have appropriate expectations in all of these areas are good candidates. Finally, be sure you thoroughly understand the procedure you'd be undergoing—the risks, the benefits, and the limitations imposed by your anatomy. Having a clear picture of what's ahead contributes to your having a realistic outlook.

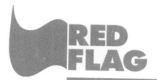
RED FLAG

Certain emotional disorders can rule out cosmetic surgery

Body dysmorphic disorder, or BDD: This is a clinically recognized mental disorder in which sufferers obsess about imagined defects in their appearance, often to such an extreme that it disrupts their daily lives. A good surgeon will not operate on someone with such a problem, but will instead refer her for counseling.

Eating disorders: People who have eating disorders often suffer from a distorted body image. Until the eating disorder has been brought under control by counseling, a good surgeon would caution against any cosmetic surgery.

Substance addiction: An addiction to any mood-altering substance or drug signifies an inability to cope with everyday problems. Again, cosmetic surgery would not be recommended until the addiction had been successfully treated in counseling.

Certain physical conditions must be addressed before having cosmetic surgery

Disorders of the heart, lung, or central nervous system could increase the risk of blood clotting.

Smoking interferes with wound healing. Most doctors will ask you to stop smoking for a time before and after your operation.

finding a doctor

Where to go for referrals

If you are a little anxious or self-conscious about asking friends and colleagues for a referral for a cosmetic surgeon, you are not alone. Many people still feel cosmetic surgery is a very private matter. Doctors and dentists are excellent referral sources. Call and ask if they know of any plastic surgeons they would recommend. Another source is your local hospital. Another is the Internet. You can log on in the privacy of your home and find out not only the names of cosmetic surgeons in your area, but also their specialty, as well as information on their education, training, and certification.

As you do your research, pay close attention to the doctor's area of specialty. Plastic surgeons are trained in many different procedures, but that doesn't mean they are good at all of them. Make sure the doctor you choose has considerable experience in the procedure you are seeking to have done. If you are not sure about what you want, make sure the doctor has experience in those areas of the body in which you are seeking improvement.

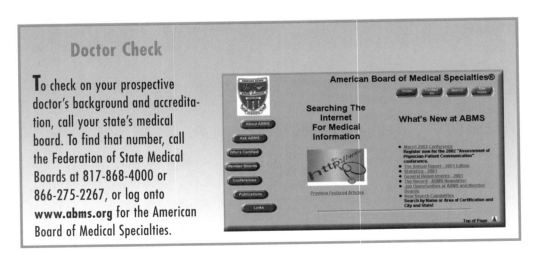

Doctor Check

To check on your prospective doctor's background and accreditation, call your state's medical board. To find that number, call the Federation of State Medical Boards at 817-868-4000 or 866-275-2267, or log onto **www.abms.org** for the American Board of Medical Specialties.

ask the experts

How important is certification?

Certification cannot be stressed enough. Ideally, you want a surgeon who's certified by the American Board of Plastic Surgery and a member of the American Society of Plastic Surgery (ASPS), the largest plastic surgery specialty organization in the world. (The Canadian equivalent is the Royal College of Physicians and Surgeons of Canada.) The ASPS has the endorsement of the American Medical Association and the American Board of Plastic Surgery, the leading accreditation organizations in the U.S. Such certification means that not only has your doctor graduated from an accredited medical school and completed a minimum of five years of general and plastic surgery residency training, but he has also passed the rigorous tests given by the board. If your doctor is not a member, that is a red flag. (For more information on boards, see page 190.) You want to avoid, say, your friendly podiatrist, who may have just taken a liposuction course over the weekend and is now offering the procedure.

Should I worry about my doctor having hospital privileges if I'm not having the procedure done in a hospital?

Before granting privileges, hospitals evaluate a surgeon's training and competency in a particular surgical procedure. If your doctor lacks hospital privileges for your type of surgery, heed the red flag and look for another surgeon. If the procedure is being performed in your doctor's office or a surgical center, check on the availability and type of lifesaving and monitoring equipment, the qualifications of the person administering your anesthesia, and other staff. You can check out the surgical facility through three agencies, which are listed on page 190.

the consultation

Interviewing your doctor

It's a good idea to see at least three doctors to get as much information as you can before you decide to undergo any procedure. Your emotional and physical health is on the line; don't go with the first doctor you see.

Note: Some plastic surgeons charge for a consultation because not only are they providing you with information about their practice and experience, but they are also evaluating your needs and offering their expertise. (Some doctors will apply that consultation fee toward any work you have done.) So come prepared with all relevant information about your health. Typically, you will be asked to fill out a form about your medical history. This is extremely important as certain health conditions may rule out cosmetic surgery or require your plastic surgeon to work with your other medical providers to address a complication first.

When you meet the doctor, she will review your medical history. Help the doctor help you: Tell her of any previous surgeries or present conditions that you have and of any medications that you take, including herbal remedies, nutritional supplements, and any psychiatric medications (anti-depressants, anti-anxiety drugs). Highlight any allergies or injuries you have or have had.

Next, the doctor will ask you to talk about your appearance concerns. A lot of people feel bashful about telling the doctor what they have in mind, but don't be. The desire to look better is not only not a crime, it's the reason you're there. The more up-front you can be, the better. A doctor cannot respond to your desires unless you make clear exactly what they are.

ask the experts

Can computer imaging show me what I could look like after surgery? And what about "before" and "after" photos?

Computer imaging can give you an idea of what you might look like after surgery, but it's not a 100% reliable forecast because of all the variables involved, such as your anatomy, skin, and healing abilities. "Before" and "after" photos should be thought of as no more than a general guide—you can't expect your results to look exactly like someone else's "after" picture. And don't forget that photos can be retouched to make the end result look better than it really was. Ask the doctor if you can talk with the patients he has photographed. Most patients are so happy with their results they are pleased to help others achieve the same.

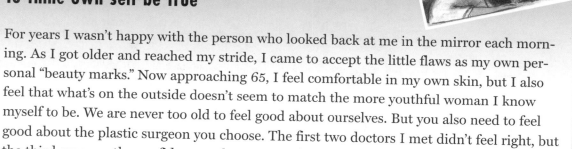

CAUTIONARY TALE

To thine own self be true

For years I wasn't happy with the person who looked back at me in the mirror each morning. As I got older and reached my stride, I came to accept the little flaws as my own personal "beauty marks." Now approaching 65, I feel comfortable in my own skin, but I also feel that what's on the outside doesn't seem to match the more youthful woman I know myself to be. We are never too old to feel good about ourselves. But you also need to feel good about the plastic surgeon you choose. The first two doctors I met didn't feel right, but the third gave me the confidence to have cosmetic surgery.

Marcy G., Philadelphia, Pennsylvania

what to ask

Come prepared with a list of smart questions

Once you are comfortable with your prospective doctor, it's time to discuss the details of your procedure, your recovery, costs, and your expectations. Don't be hesitant. Remember, your health and well-being are at stake.

The Procedure

- What procedures are there for the outcome I am seeking? What are the pros and cons of each? Which do you recommend?

- What, if any, are my nonsurgical options? How would you compare surgical versus nonsurgical treatments?

- How long have you been performing this procedure? How many have you done this year? How often do you do it? What are your specific qualifications and training in the procedure I'm considering?

- Can you show me "before" and "after" photos and/or computer imaging of your recent work on patients who had concerns similar to my own? Can I call some of your patients and talk to them about the procedure?

- What complications are most common with this procedure, and how frequent are they? If there is a complication, is it resolvable? Will you repeat or correct a procedure if I am not happy with the outcome? If so, do you cover the costs or do I?

- How long will the procedure take? What technique will you be using? Can you describe how it works? How does it compare to other possible techniques? Is this the only technique you do or is it the one most appropriate for me and why?

- Will I have to stop smoking and taking some of my medications or supplements both before and after the treatment? For how long?

Facilities and Staff

■ Where will the procedure take place? Is the facility affiliated with a hospital? Is local or general anesthesia to be used? In general, how long might I be under?

■ Will a board-certified anesthesiologist be present? If not, who will administer the anesthetic? If you don't perform the entire surgery yourself, who will be assisting? What are her qualifications?

Recovery

■ Will a registered nurse be present during my recovery? For a more extensive cosmetic surgery procedure, do you have an affiliation with a facility and/or nursing program for post-operative care? How long is the recovery period? How much post-operative bruising, swelling, and pain can I expect? What type of post-operative care will I need? How long will I need to take time off from work? What scars will this procedure leave? Will I be able to hide them?

Costs

■ How much will the procedure cost? Do you require payment up front? Can you give me an estimate of the total cost, including fees for the facility, medications, and post-operative follow-up appointments?

Special Concerns

■ If I am considering more than one procedure, should I have them done at the same time? What are the pros and cons to doing so?

■ Have you ever had your malpractice insurance coverage denied, revoked, or suspended?

Expectations

■ Are my desired results realistic? How long will the results last?

the cost

What your insurance will—and won't—pay for

There is a body of research that tells us that not only are attractive people seen in a more favorable light, they also receive preferential treatment. Since appearance seems to matter so much in our society, it would seem to be in people's best interest to do what they can to enhance it. Unfortunately, insurance companies have not yet bought into this thinking.

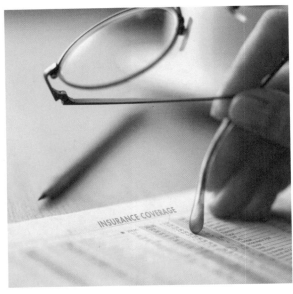

Insurers are fully prepared to cover reconstructive procedures to correct features damaged by trauma (such as an accident), disease, or congenital defects (those present at birth) that interfere with normal body functions and thus are deemed medically necessary. Insurers will not cover procedures that you choose to have done solely to enhance your appearance (known as **elective procedures** in insuranceland). That is why you or your doctor should check with your insurance carrier about the extent of your coverage before you undergo surgery. Be prepared to pay the bill yourself. Often, plastic surgeons request a portion of their payment before they operate.

Cosmetic surgery costs range from several hundred to several thousand dollars, depending on various factors: the complexity of the procedure to be performed, the type of facility in which the surgery will take place (a hospital, a doctor's office, or a surgical facility), which anesthetic will be used, any post-op care or products you may require, and the going rate for the procedure in your geographic location. Whatever the cost, it is never a good idea to bargain-shop—your surgeon's experience and training should not be things you compromise on for a dollar.

ask the experts

When will an insurance carrier cover the costs?

If your insurer decides that your procedure is for relief of medical problems and not simply for cosmetic improvement, you may be covered, at least in part. Before your treatment, have your doctor submit pre-authorization material to your insurer for review. Some examples of what may be covered: breast implants for those who have had a mastectomy, hair replacement due to loss of hair from burns or trauma, or eyelid surgery if droopy lids interfere with vision.

What are examples of some costs for cosmetic surgery procedures?

Surgeons' fees alone range from $4,000 to $14,000 or more for a facelift; $2,000 to $7,000 for liposuction; $3,000 to $6,000 for breast implants; $3,000 to $9,000 for a hair transplant; $2,500 to $6,500 for a nose reduction; and $2,000 to $7,000 for upper/lower eyelid surgery. (In the following chapters, you will find the fee ranges for each type of procedure.)

Get the breakdown and total of the costs spelled out in writing beforehand. Clarify early on whether your form of treatment will require multiple visits and, if so, at what rate. Many doctors charge for the initial consultation, but some do not, so ask about this when you set up that appointment. Also, some doctors offer package pricing for multiple procedures performed at the same time in the same setting. Ask about combined treatment pricing if you're considering having, say, liposuction on your hips along with an eyelid tuck.

Your Bill

- Your surgeon's fee
- Pre-operative physical and blood work
- Operating facility fee
- Anesthesiologist's fee
- Costs for any medical supplies (surgical garments)
- Medications or any other post-surgical accommodations (private-duty nursing)
- Possible touch-up treatments
- Post-operative checkups

now what do I do?

Answers to common questions

Who is the typical person seeking cosmetic surgery?

Most men and women who have cosmetic surgery are no different from individuals who don't—they're not known to be more depressed or to have lower self-esteem than the rest of the population. Typically, those considering cosmetic surgery spend considerable time (on average six years, one study found) thinking it through before finally doing it. They are also known to make a greater investment in health and fitness in general, and many view cosmetic surgery as an extension of, say, going to the gym.

Is there any one factor that rules out having cosmetic surgery?

Smoking can be a deal-breaker. Because it decreases blood flow, it greatly increases the likelihood of surgical complications. It can delay healing and cause tissue loss and scarring. Some surgeons refuse to operate on smokers; others will proceed if the smoker stops for several weeks before and after the procedure. While such abstinence may help minimize the risks, the nicotine withdrawal could make your recovery more difficult.

What is the best age to have cosmetic surgery?

It depends on the procedure. For certain surgeries, such as a nose reshaping, patients need to wait until the nose is fully matured, usually around age 17. On the other hand, otoplasty (surgery to correct protruding ears) can be performed on kids as young as 5, when the ear is fully developed. Some hair replacement procedures will not be very effective until most of your hair loss has occurred—perhaps well into your 30s. A facelift is not recommended until you have reached your mid-40s.

Will I have visible scars from a procedure?

Your surgeon will try to hide incisions, and thus scars, in the hairline and the normal creases of your skin. Some areas, such as your ankles, are not suitable for surgery involving incisions because there would be no place to conceal a scar. Unfortunately, some procedures are prone to result in problem scarring—although that is a risk with any surgery.

Should I tell my other healthcare providers that I've had a cosmetic surgery procedure?

Yes, you should always give your doctors your complete medical history, including any type of surgery you've undergone, whether it was performed in a hospital or an outpatient facility, and whether you were given general or local anesthesia.

Now where do I go?!

CONTACTS

American Society
of Plastic Surgeons
www.plasticsurgery.org
847-228-9900

American Society
for Aesthetic Plastic Surgery
www.surgery.org
212-921-0500

American Academy of Facial Plastic
and Reconstructive Surgery
www.aafprs.org
800-332-FACE

ADDITIONAL INFORMATION

Everything You Ever Wanted to Know About Cosmetic Surgery but Couldn't Afford to Ask
By Alan Gaynor, M.D.

The Smart Woman's Guide to Plastic Surgery: Essential Information from a Female Plastic Surgeon
By Jean M. Loftus, M.D.

Plastic Surgery: What You Need to Know—Before, During, and After
By Richard A. Marfuggi, M.D.

Chapter 2

Skin Care Smarts

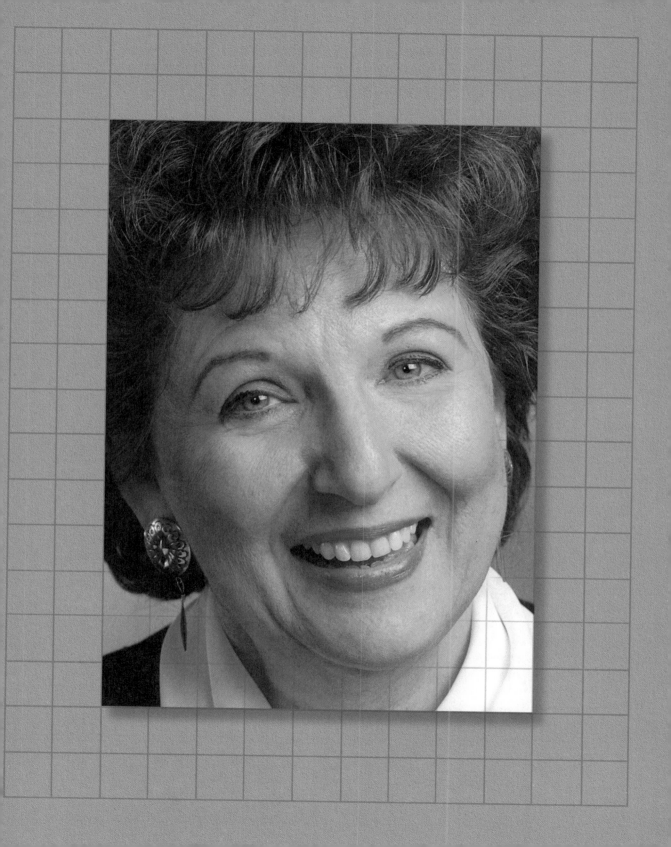

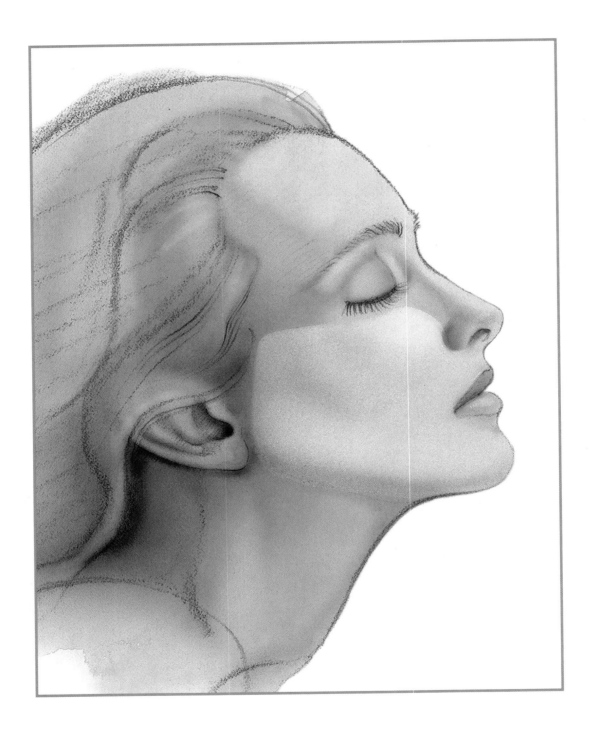

As the largest organ of the body, the skin has a huge job. It must protect us from the outside world—UV rays from the sun, variable climates, and pollution—to say nothing of internal assaults in the form of poor health habits, inadequate nutrition, and illness. From simple regimens to an arsenal of high-powered treatments, dermatologists and plastic surgeons can do much to restore lost luster to your skin.

skin care basics

Nonsurgical care for your skin

The good news is that while age, stress, sun exposure, and pollution will all inevitably take a toll on your skin, you can slow that process with proper care. Here's a primer on what you need and why:

Soap A mild soap to clean the skin of dirt and other surface debris. People with dry skin should use a "superfatted" soap bar that contains ingredients such as olive oil or lanolin.

Exfoliants Products containing exfoliants help clear away dry, flaky skin and unclog skin pores. They leave your face feeling smoother and softer. The most effective exfoliant is Retin-A, a derivative of vitamin A. Some over-the-counter products now contain retinols or other vitamin A derivatives, but only in small amounts. For a more dramatic result, consult a dermatologist, who can prescribe stronger versions.

Occlusives These products (petroleum jelly, cocoa butter, mineral oil) trap the skin's moisture without being absorbed.

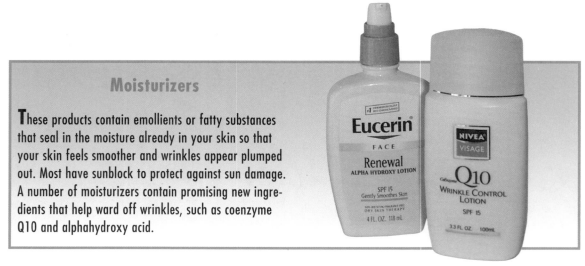

Moisturizers

These products contain emollients or fatty substances that seal in the moisture already in your skin so that your skin feels smoother and wrinkles appear plumped out. Most have sunblock to protect against sun damage. A number of moisturizers contain promising new ingredients that help ward off wrinkles, such as coenzyme Q10 and alphahydroxy acid.

ask the experts

What is an effective daily skin care regimen?

In the morning Wash your face with a very mild soap in warm water (hot is drying and cold won't open the pores). Pat dry, leaving your face slightly wet (don't rub it dry with a towel). Apply moisturizer while your face is still damp, as this will help lock in extra moisture. Then rub on sunscreen (see the next page). Finally, apply makeup. (Put on the sunscreen *before* the moisturizer if your skin is already dry.)

At night Wash your face in warm water (not hot or cold) using a mild exfoliant such as one containing retinol or glycolic acid.

Warning Stay away from toner and astringent. These products are usually made with alcohol; their purpose is to get rid of excess oiliness. Most dermatologists advise against them since they can dry skin too much.

Skin Types

There are five skin types: normal, dry, oily, combination, and sensitive. What type of skin you have is determined by genetics and your lifestyle. For example, smoking dries the skin; so does excessive use of alcohol. Combination skin means dry in parts, oily in others—typically the forehead and the nose. Using the wrong skin care product can actually harm your skin, so check with a dermatologist for advice about what's best for you.

sunblock

The number one face-saver

Nothing will age your skin faster than exposure to the sun. What exactly does sunlight do to the skin? The UV rays in sunlight gradually degrade the collagen and elastic tissues in skin that keep it smooth and firm. That's why over time sun exposure results in wrinkles and sagging skin. UV rays also stimulate the skin to create freckles and age spots. And these rays can damage DNA, which in the worst case can trigger skin cancers.

To protect against this damage, you need to block out the harmful UV rays. There are two types to shield against: **ultraviolet-A** (UVA) and **ultraviolet-B** (UVB). Both do serious damage: UVA is regarded as the main culprit in wrinkling, leathery skin and other aspects of aging skin. UVB, coupled with UVA, can cause various types of skin cancer.

Your best defense against all harmful rays is to wear protective clothing and a wide-brimmed hat, and apply sunblock frequently. The protection factor in sunblock or sunscreen is calculated for UVB rays based on how long the skin takes to turn red without such protection. For example, if it takes 20 minutes without protection, using an SPF 15 sunscreen should stave off reddening 15 times longer—for about 5 hours. But if you start to burn in only 10 minutes, you would get only $2^{1/2}$ hours of protection from that same SPF 15. Because the protection can vary with the individual (and how well and how often she applies sunblock), many experts believe you should use an SPF of 30, and apply it every 2 hours, plus after being in the water to be safe.

ask the experts

How much sunscreen should I put on?

People often skimp on the amount of sunscreen they put on. You need to apply it generously and frequently for it to be effective: a tablespoonful for the face and a liberal amount to cover the entire body. Apply sunscreen 30 minutes before going out in the sun, to give it time to bind with the skin.

What kinds of sunscreen are there?

There are two types: chemical and physical. Chemical sunscreens protect you from the sun by absorbing the ultraviolet and visible rays, while physical sunscreens reflect, scatter, or block these rays. Chemical sunscreens are absorbed by the body; physical sunscreens are not—they remain on top of the skin. Be sure to buy a product that protects against both UVA and UVB rays, regardless of its form. And throw away last year's sunblock since the protective properties diminish with time, especially when exposed to heat.

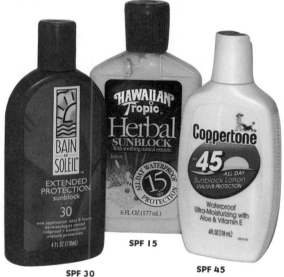

SPF 30

SPF 15

SPF 45

What's the best sun protection available for swimmers?

Water-resistant sunscreen is available. It is effective for about 1½ hours before needing to be reapplied. If you go in the water, however, reapply it immediately after coming out, no matter how briefly you were wet.

Note: Because water reflects sunlight, you could be exposed to more UV rays than if you were lying on a towel. For that reason swimmers should use an SPF of at least 30.

SPF stands for sun protection factor. It measures how long you can stay out in the sun without protection before getting a sunburn from UVB rays. Most dermatologists recommend an SPF of 15 or higher, depending on your activity and special needs.

seeing a dermatologist

What innovations in this field can do for you

Over-the-counter skin products like moisturizers and exfoliants can help give your skin a fresher, more youthful feel. But they can't get rid of wrinkles, nor erase the harsher evidence of aging skin, such as **dyschromia**, which includes early brown spots, such as **lentigines** (also known as liver spots), dots, and freckles. As you get older, you'll see lines at the outer corners of the eyes (crow's feet), crepe-like appearance beneath the eyes, and **keratoses** (scaly red spots). For help with these and other skin issues, you need to see a dermatologist (a doctor who specializes in the care and treatment of the skin).

There are four basic types of procedures that can help with aging skin: injections, peels, dermabrasion, and lasers. (All but lasers are discussed in this chapter; see the next chapter for laser treatment of the skin.) Some of these treatments require a month or so of preparation under your dermatologist's supervision before they can be done.

Not all treatments are appropriate for everyone. And some procedures are quite intense. You want to be sure you're in the hands of a qualified dermatologist or plastic surgeon. (See pages 15 and 190 for more on credentials.)

ask the experts

How do I find a dermatologist in my area?

Ask family and friends for referrals. Another great referral source is your family doctor or dentist. Call and ask if they know of any dermatologists they would recommend. Another source is your local hospital. Still another is the American Academy of Dermatology; contact them at **www.aad.org** or call 888-462-DERM.

Who would I go to for skin treatment, a dermatologist or a plastic surgeon?

Dermatologists deal with all manner of skin care, including such cosmetic treatments as skin peels, injections, lasers, and Botox (read more about each of these treatments in this chapter and the one that follows). Plastic surgeons can also do many of these, but are more specialized in cosmetic (and reconstructive) surgery.

Can I go to a spa for a facial peel?

Yes, but it's not advised. You don't want to put your face in untrained hands. The importance of qualifications, training, and experience cannot be overstated. You want a trained medical professional treating you, not someone who spent a weekend learning about facial peels. To check on your prospective doctor's background and accreditation, call your state's medical board. To find that number, call the Federation of State Medical Boards at 817-868-4000 or 866-275-2267, or log onto **www.abms.org** for the American Board of Medical Specialties.

botox

Stop fine lines and crow's feet in their tracks

After a certain age, we develop wrinkles in the upper third of the face due to years of using the muscles there when we laugh, frown, etc. Crow's feet around the eyes, horizontal lines in the forehead, and deepening vertical lines between the brows begin to appear. In the past the wrinkles could only be reduced with lasers or a facelift, but an ingenious medical discovery has come to the rescue. Doctors found that injections of botulinum toxin, or **Botox**, a substance used to stop persistent twitching of eye muscles, also made the patient's forehead wrinkles disappear. Botox paralyzes the underlying muscle it's injected into, so the line or wrinkle that muscle causes simply flattens out.

The Botox treatment itself takes 5 to 20 minutes. Roughly a thimbleful of Botox is injected per area—how much is needed depends on the size of the muscle being treated. In general, 3 shots per eye are needed to treat crow's feet, 4 to 6 injections are used for between-brow lines (where the muscle is thicker and deeper) and 6 to 8 are needed for the forehead. Note: Men often require more Botox than women because their facial muscles are thicker.

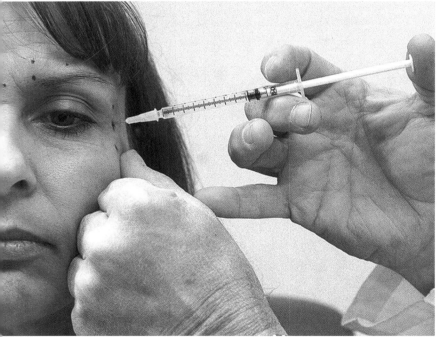

Your doctor will have you contract the muscle in your forehead so he can see where the lines appear and mark the spot. Then a numbing cream or an ice pack may be applied to the site to prepare it for the injection.

ask the experts

How safe is Botox?

Botox is made from the toxin that causes botulism, a severe form of food poisoning. Don't worry, you can't get it from an injection. (To get botulism, you need to eat food that has been tainted with the botulinum toxin.) While you can have a bruise for 24 to 36 hours, the real risks are a droopy eyelid or **ptosis**, which is a droopy forehead or brow. Note: Botox naturally wears off, so this would return to normal in 3 to 4 months.

How much should I do and how long will the effects of Botox last?

For the initial procedure, confine the treatment to just one area, to make sure you have no adverse reactions to the Botox and are satisfied with the results. You can redo an area 2 weeks later if you're not satisfied. Though everyone responds differently, results typically last 3 to 4 months, when most people go back for another round of injections. Often, the results become cumulative—the more you do it, the better the outcome. That's because the muscles become less activated over time, so it will take fewer treatments each year to achieve the same result.

What happens after the treatment? What is recovery like?

Other than applying some ice at first, you can go right back to work. Later, when you go home, it's a good idea to contract or flex the facial muscles to integrate the Botox more quickly into the treated area. You'll be advised not to bend over for the first few hours to decrease the risk of the brow or forehead drooping. It takes between 3 and 7 days before you'll see the results. Sometimes it takes 10 days to 2 weeks, depending on the area.

FEES

Botox

Doctors' fees are between $300 and $600 per area treated. For the entire upper third of the face, the cost can range from $1,000 to $1,500.

collagen

Help for laugh lines, thinning lips, and more

Over the years, among the most prominent wrinkles we develop are laugh lines, those deep lines that start at the base of each nostril and go around the mouth and almost down to the chin. They are also called the **nasolabial folds**. The reason for the deep creases—besides gravity—is a loss of **collagen** and fat beneath the skin. (Collagen is the fibrous protein in the connective tissue that supports and strengthens the skin.) Collagen is also lost in the lips, which is why they begin to look thinner and the lower lip droops.

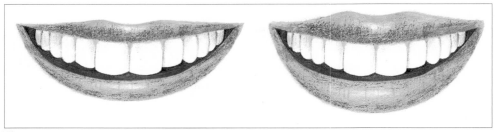

The lips can be treated in just 30 minutes; you can have this done during your lunch hour.

To address these signs of aging, as well as fine lines on the cheek, there is **soft-tissue augmentation**, the most common method being collagen injection. The most popular filling material is purified bovine collagen, derived from the skin of cows. The lips and nasolabial folds can be treated during a single, half-hour visit that typically involves 2 or 3 syringes of collagen. These injections tend to be more uncomfortable than those for Botox (see page 34), especially in the lips, so a numbing cream is applied first. Because the syringe also contains an anesthetic, the injections gradually become less painful during the treatment.

ask the experts

How much does precision count when a doctor is injecting collagen?

Where the doctor injects the collagen is where it's going to stay. If he is not precise, you will see a bump for months. If the collagen is injected too close to the skin's surface, it will cause a lump. It can also be accidentally injected into a blood vessel, resulting in uneven skin tone and other complications.

What are the risks associated with collagen?

Bruising and an allergic reaction are the most common. If an allergy develops, it could result in lumps and bumps on your face that can last between 6 and 12 months. About 3% of adults are allergic to collagen. Therefore, you'll need to take two skin patch tests about a month before treatment. While this will reduce the potential for a reaction, you may still develop an allergy to collagen later. Collagen injections are not recommended for those with allergies to beef or other bovine products, or those with an autoimmune disease, such as lupus.

What happens after having the injections? What is recovery like?

You might be a bit swollen and red, but you should be able to return to work immediately. Applying an ice pack for about 10 to 15 minutes should reduce the swelling and redness.

Can collagen and Botox be combined in one visit?

Absolutely. Your doctor may first inject the collagen into the lips or nasolabial folds, and apply an ice pack for 10 minutes. Then he'll inject Botox into your forehead and apply an ice pack.

How long does the effect of a collagen injection last?

Results typically last about 3 to 4 months for laugh lines; lips about a month.

FEES

Collagen

The price of a single syringe of collagen, which is the standard unit, starts at $400. The total cost will depend on how much you need. For example, one syringe may be enough to add minor plump to the lips and laugh lines. On the other hand, treating very deep wrinkles could cost more than $1,000.

fat and filler injections

Alternatives to collagen for plumping deep creases

Fat and Filler Injections

The cost of fat injection varies. For small fat removal and storage, the fee ranges from $1,000 to $2,000. If a bigger liposuction procedure is performed along with a fat transfer, that cost can more than double—depending on the volume removed. Other filler injectables cost around $250 to $500 per syringe, depending on the material.

Materials other than collagen can be used to fill in those not-so-funny laugh lines and plump up thinning lips. For example, your doctor can take fat from your own body—usually the belly, hips, or thighs—and transfer it to your face. The fat is "harvested" with a syringe or liposuction (see page 138). After making a small incision in the area, your doctor vacuums out what amounts to at least a handful of fat and closes the area. The fat is separated out into microdroplets, which are then injected into your face. The harvesting of the fat can take up to an hour; the injections, about 30 minutes. A bonus: You can't be allergic to your own fat.

If you're not keen on the idea of having fat harvested from your own body (you can't use fat from someone else), you can opt for other kinds of soft-tissue fillers. **Cymetra** is made from ground-up human tissue that has undergone viral and bacterial screening. There are also other, not-yet-FDA-approved filling substances, such as the hyaluronic acid-based gels **Hylaform** and **Restylane**. While all of these collagen-like products are believed to last longer than conventional bovine collagen, you will still need periodic, ongoing injections to maintain results.

ask the experts

Can fat be stored for later use?

Yes. Harvested fat can be frozen and stored by your doctor for up to a year.

What are the risk and recovery issues with fat injections?

Human fat is much thicker and more viscous than bovine or human collagen, so it requires a larger needle to inject it. That can result in significant bruising. Swelling can last for anywhere from 10 minutes to 2 days to 2 months, depending on the technique appropriate for your problem. Perhaps the worst—and fortunately, rarest—risk with any injectable material is **occlusion**, where the material clogs up or pushes up against a blood vessel and causes decreased blood flow to an area, which can result in scarring.

How long does fat last?

The longevity of fat is widely variable, lasting from months to years. Studies show that while some of the injected fat always dissipates, 30% to 70% survives from each injection, depending on the technique. Thus, the more often you have fat injected, the longer lasting your results.

Are there any other places you can inject the fat once you remove it for the transfer to my lips?

Your hands and cheeks are great areas for fat injections, which act like padding under a carpet. Few things give away our age faster than our hands, despite a facelift or other age-fighting procedures.

mild face peels

One way to diminish fine lines and even out skin tone

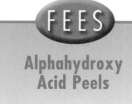

FEES

Alphahydroxy Acid Peels

Doctors' fees for acid peels range from $100 to $250 per treatment.

If filler injections aren't for you or they're not the real answer to your problem, resurfacing is the next option. The most common technique uses certain chemicals that are painted on the face. These chemicals peel away the top, damaged layer of the skin to allow a fresh new layer to emerge. Mild resurfacing can reduce wrinkles, erase blemishes, correct uneven skin tone (**dyschromia**), and clear up some minor acne scarring.

Your doctor will most likely start you off with an at-home topical regimen. He will prescribe a mild exfoliating agent such as Retin-A or glycolic acid to be used at night, starting with low concentrations and gradually increasing the strength. In high concentrations, these agents will peel away the top layer of skin.

For more extensive rejuvenation, your doctor will use **alphahydroxy acid (AHA) peels**. These are stronger concentrations of glycolic, lactic, and fruit acids. This in-office procedure calls for your skin to be cleansed, after which the acid is applied to your face for a few moments and then washed off. (Because chemical peels leave your skin more sensitive to the sun, it's imperative that you use sunscreen every day.)

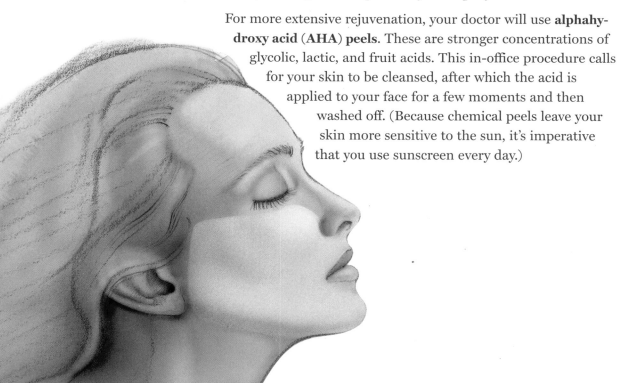

ask the experts

How long does it last?

Peels require a series of about six treatments, typically performed on a monthly basis, and there is very little recovery time. Mild peels will yield subtle results, though over time they will give your skin a healthy glow.

What are the risks associated with this procedure?

Acid peels can cause stinging, redness, dryness, or irritation. Or you could have an allergic reaction to the product. In rare cases, you could also get a burn or infection, or even suffer scarring.

What is the difference between what the doctor will apply to my skin and what I can buy over the counter?

The products you get over the counter are very low dose and low concentration. The higher the concentration, the more effective the product can be. But it will also be more irritating, which is why only your doctor can administer it.

Microdermabrasion

Another office-based resurfacing method is **microdermabrasion**, which is appropriate for someone with a bit more discoloration and fine lines. Here, a small wand filled with tiny particles gently **abrades**, or scrapes away, the damaged surface of the skin, while a vacuum tube applies suction; this mild abrasion stimulates new cell growth. Like the peel, this procedure goes deeper into the skin than at-home treatment. Microdermabrasion is similar in cost to the AHA peel. (See page 46 for more on dermabrasion.)

stronger peels

Medium-depth peels treat lines and skin-tone variations that demand more

While mild chemical peels work on the uppermost layer of skin, called the **epidermis**, more serious facial lines and pigment variations may require your doctor to work deeper into the skin. **Medium-depth peels**, known as **trichloroacetic acid** (**TCA**) **peels**, are designed to work on the next layer of skin, known as the **dermis**.

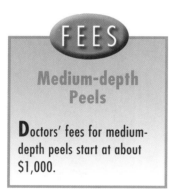

FEES

Medium-depth Peels

Doctors' fees for medium-depth peels start at about $1,000.

Medium-depth chemical peels are much more invasive than the milder alphahydroxy peels (see previous page). Your doctor is essentially taking an acid and applying it to your skin. While no sedation is necessary, the procedure is uncomfortable. For that reason, your doctor may administer a local anesthetic to certain areas.

For the procedure, your eyes and lips are first covered for protection. Then your skin is cleansed with alcohol to remove surface oils. Next, TCA is painted over the entire skin surface. Your doctor will feather the acid into your hairline and a little under the chin, so the results will blend in and not leave an obvious cut-off point around your face. In addition to the face, this type of peel can be used on the neck and other areas of the body. The procedure takes 30 to 60 minutes, depending on the extent of the area being treated.

A medium-depth peel is very hard on the skin, requiring at least 7 to 10 days of healing. This is yet another reason to have only a qualified doctor treat you (see page 14). Usually only one treatment is required, but you may need more than one TCA peel to achieve the desired result.

ask the experts

Who is the best candidate for a medium-depth peel?

The ideal candidate is an older woman who is showing moderate signs of aging with a lot of freckles and static lines—fine wrinkles caused by fat loss and gravity, not muscle movement. Static lines are best treated with collagen or other injectables. People who have had a lot of sun damage, or who were heavy smokers, make good candidates because, typically, they have more lines than injectables can handle. Darker-skinned people are well suited to this type of treatment.

If I've already had a medium-depth peel, is it possible to just redo one area?

Often a line will come back, or you may want a bit more done in one spot. Your doctor can treat that specific area; she doesn't have to redo the entire face. This is true for all skin resurfacing procedures.

What are the risks associated with medium-depth peels?

Your skin could become lighter or darker in certain areas. Acid peels can cause stinging, redness, dryness, or irritation. Or you could have an allergic reaction to the product. In rare cases you could also get a burn or infection, or even suffer scarring.

What happens after the treatment? What is recovery like?

You won't have to wear a dressing or mask, but you will need to apply emollients (creams and oils that soothe the skin). The next day you will be swollen. Because your face has in effect sustained a relatively deep burn from the acid, your skin will look brown and begin to peel and scab. Your doctor will see you repeatedly to make sure you're healing properly. Your face will continue to peel for about a week, and you'll be out of commission for a week to 10 days. For several months, in order to protect the newly forming layers of skin, you will have to wear sunscreen and a wide-brimmed hat to shield your face outdoors at all times.

the strongest peel

Powerful phenol peels for deep facial lines and more

The **phenol peel** is best for fair-skinned people in their 50s or 60s who have significant sun damage, very deep lines, and blotchy areas that won't respond to less invasive peels. The phenol peel goes deeper into the skin, to the layer safest to penetrate, and delivers a rather profound insult to the skin. However, the cosmetic results are dramatic and long-lasting (typically, this is a one-time procedure).

A phenol peel takes from 1 to 2 hours. Because it results in a very deep injury to your skin, your doctor will do regional nerve blocks to anesthetize specific facial areas and will give you sedation. Your skin is cleansed and alcohol is applied to remove surface oils. Then the phenol-based solution is painted on your face, starting with the forehead and onto the ear and beneath the chin, feathering into the hairline.

The solution is left on each area for 15 to 30 minutes to allow the body to absorb the chemical before the next area is painted. Because the phenol is absorbed, there's a potential for it to damage the heart, kidneys, and liver. While these peels don't have to be done in a hospital, they do require heart monitoring (during and after the procedure). If you have a history of heart disease, this treatment may not be appropriate for you. You will be closely watched for any heart problems or discomfort.

Note: Because the skin often gets lighter following treatment, deep peels are not recommended for people of color.

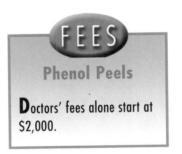

FEES

Phenol Peels

Doctors' fees alone start at $2,000.

ask the experts

What risks are associated with this type of treatment?

Deep peels are very caustic and cause significant injury to the skin. You will need to be monitored, because the deeper you go into the skin, the greater the potential for harm. In addition, there is a risk of adverse reaction to the phenol. Other potential complications, while rare, are scarring, burns, and infection. If you're prone to cold sores, the treatment may stir up the herpes virus that causes them. And because this peel will often render your new skin unable to tan, you will need to be conscientious about avoiding sun exposure and using sunblock.

What happens after the treatment? What is recovery like?

Your face will be swollen when you leave the doctor's office and become more swollen that night and for the next couple of days. During that time you will likely be on a liquid diet and not able to talk very much. Because the procedure basically burns your skin, your face will turn red and you might need to wear a bandage mask for 2 days. Your doctor will see you nearly every day for 2 weeks for follow-up. You will have to refrain from strenuous activity for 2 weeks or more.

CAUTIONARY TALE

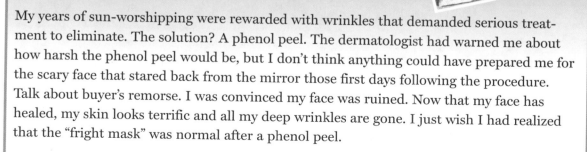

Be prepared

My years of sun-worshipping were rewarded with wrinkles that demanded serious treatment to eliminate. The solution? A phenol peel. The dermatologist had warned me about how harsh the phenol peel would be, but I don't think anything could have prepared me for the scary face that stared back from the mirror those first days following the procedure. Talk about buyer's remorse. I was convinced my face was ruined. Now that my face has healed, my skin looks terrific and all my deep wrinkles are gone. I just wish I had realized that the "fright mask" was normal after a phenol peel.

Betsy S., Long Beach Island, New Jersey

attack your acne

Dermabrasion can smooth away those acne scars

Long after the embarrassing adolescent condition has faded, acne leaves its sufferers with scars, usually in the form of ice-pick scars (deep, narrow crevices) or other **atrophic** scars (depressed, crater-like areas). **Dermabrasion**, which is a controlled abrading, or sanding down, of the top layers of skin, is the most effective treatment for acne scarring.

Your doctor first cleans and anesthetizes the skin. Then she mechanically sands down the skin using a rotary instrument to remove the damaged tissue. The treatment takes 2 to 3 hours, and can be quite bloody. It will take a while for the skin to fully recover; during the healing process the skin remodels itself into a smoother, much-improved appearance.

Another treatment option, particularly if your acne is not yet under control, or if you have atrophic dish-shaped and rolling-hill acne scars, is **laser resurfacing** (see the following chapter for much more on this subject). Depending on the type of laser used, this treatment yields a 25% to 70% improvement with a minimum of four treatments. And whereas dermabrasion can safely be used only on the face, lasers can also be used for acne scarring on the neck, chest, and back—areas that tend to be difficult to treat.

For ice-pick scars, laser peels are generally done in combination with punch incisions or punch grafts, in which the doctor cuts out the little scars and sews them up, or inserts a small graft of skin taken from elsewhere on your body, to improve the overall result. Again, multiple treatments are necessary to achieve the best result.

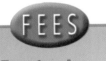

FEES

Treating Acne

Doctors' fees for dermabrasion range from $1,500 to $3,000 per treatment. Laser fees range from $2,000 to $7,000.

ask the experts

What results should I expect with dermabrasion?

In general, you will see improvement with only one treatment, but to achieve the best results with dermabrasion or laser resurfacing, multiple treatments may be necessary. Don't expect to end up with perfectly smooth skin, though it should be greatly improved.

Can I fill in my acne-covered skin with synthetic material?

A variety of soft-tissue filling materials—bovine collagen, collagen-related fillers, even your own fat (see previous pages)—can be injected in small quantities below the surface of the skin to elevate atrophic, or depressed, scars (this will not work for ice-pick scars). A filling material will not change the color of the scar, but will raise it so that it's level with the rest of your skin, smoothing out the area. There is, however, a risk of overfilling, which can make the scarred area look worse.

What about using chemical peels on my acne?

In most cases, dermabrasion or lasers work best to remove the acne-scarred skin. However, mild, medium, and deep peels (see previous pages) may be suitable for your acne, depending on its severity and extent. Consult with your doctor to determine the appropriate treatment.

What about risk and recovery issues with dermabrasion?

Following dermabrasion, you will feel as if you have an extremely bad sunburn. You'll be quite uncomfortable and may need pain medication. Your skin will be raw and then crusty for the first few days. After the crust is gone you can apply makeup for camouflage. You will feel better within 7 to 10 days, after which you can return to work. Your skin will be pink for several weeks, and you'll have to protect your face from the sun for several months after treatment.

now what do I do?

Answers to common questions

I have melasma. Is there any hope for my ridding myself of this discoloration?

Melasma, the most common and most difficult-to-treat skin discoloration, appears as brown marks on the face and typically occurs during the hormonal changes of pregnancy. Likewise, some women get these marks from taking birth control pills. Older women on hormone replacement therapy can develop melasma-like brown blotches on their arms. Other times, melasma occurs for no apparent reason. Superficial melasma, which is within the top layer of skin, is treated with bleaching agents as well as exfoliation, which can include creams, peels, or microdermabrasion. (See the previous pages for information about each of these treatments.) Lasers can also be used. Topical vitamin C has also been shown to decrease pigmentation. If the pigment is in deeper layers of skin, a combination of treatments will likely be called for and can take months. And the strategy may not work.

Should I avoid sun exposure after a cosmetic skin procedure?

Many of the skin-smoothing techniques uncover layers of skin that should not be exposed to the sun. As they heal over several months, always use sunblock and wear a wide-brimmed hat. If you have resurfacing done around the eyes, you should also wear sunglasses that have 100% filters for UVA and UVB rays.

I hate my freckles. What can I do about them?

To eliminate both light and moderate freckling, which is due to the sun (people are not born with freckles), your doctor will likely start you out on topical creams, bleaches, and exfoliants. Peels and microdermabrasion are the next step, if necessary, and then lasers. Multiple treatments may be necessary if you have a lot of freckles.

Should I have a facelift before I do any skin resurfacing?

Skin resurfacing can seem to give you a mini-facelift, but it won't fix sagging skin, which needs to be cut away with a facelift. It's not uncommon to have a facelift followed by a skin-smoothing or resurfacing treatment to erase crow's feet and other lines not remedied by a facelift. (For more on the facelift, see page 176.)

What is a "lunchtime procedure"?

Any walk-in/walk-out skin treatment performed in a doctor's office that can be done during your lunch hour (or which takes an hour or less) and leaves you looking presentable is regarded as a "lunchtime procedure." This includes Botox and collagen injections, various laser treatments, and mild facial peels.

Now where do I go?!

CONTACTS

American Academy of Dermatology
www.aad.org
888-462-DERM

American Society
for Dermatologic Surgery
www.asds-net.org
800-441-ASDS

American Society
of Plastic Surgeons
www.plasticsurgery.org
888-475-2784

American Society
for Aesthetic Plastic Surgery
www.surgery.org
888-272-7711

American Academy of Facial Plastic and
Reconstructive Surgery
www.aafprs.org
800-332-FACE

ADDITIONAL INFORMATION

U.S. Food and Drug Administration
www.fda.gov

Cosmetic Surgery News
www.cosmeticsurgery-news.com

Cosmetic Surgery & Skin Care News
www.cosmetic-surgery-news.com

Chapter 3

Laser Resurfacing

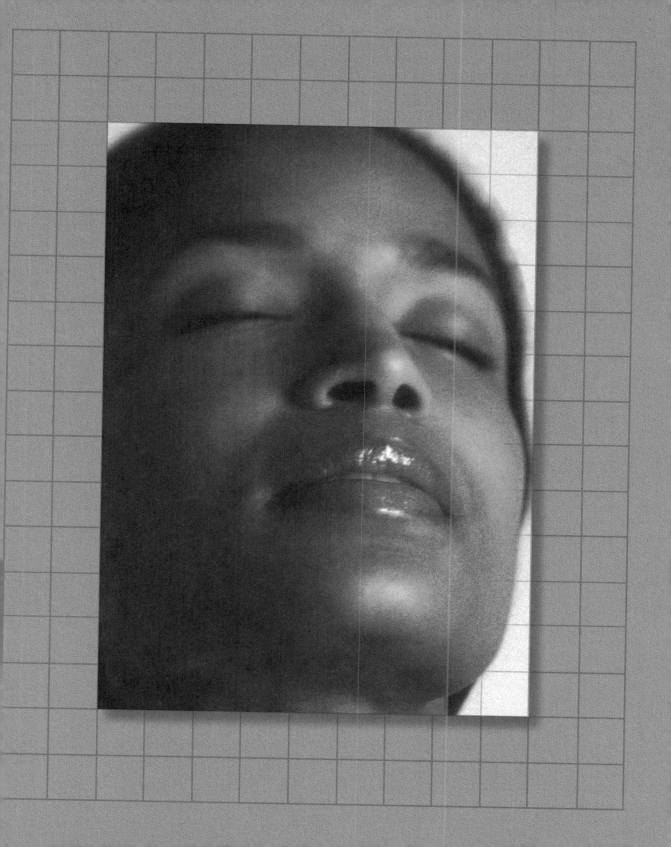

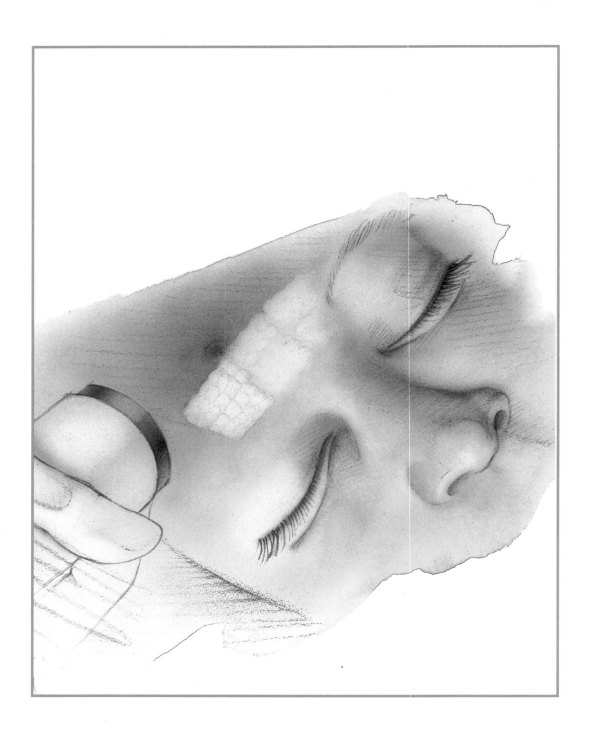

The wonder of the skin is how self-renewing it is. A sunburn is repaired in a matter of days; deep wounds heal over in a few weeks. Cosmetic surgeons have found a way to harness this ever-revitalizing aspect of skin to beautify it as well. Laser resurfacing removes the top layer of skin to permit a new, smoother layer to emerge.

what is laser resurfacing?

An alternative to chemicals for facial rejuvenation

Lasers use a beam of light energy to vaporize damaged surface skin at specific and controlled levels. (**Ablative** lasers such as the CO_2 laser remove the top layer of the skin, while **nonablative** lasers leave the top layer intact.) As the laser passes over the skin, it heats the skin, causing the **collagen** (the fibrous protein in the connective tissue that supports and strengthens the skin) to shrink and contract, thereby tightening the skin. Lasers also stimulate new collagen growth to replace the damaged tissue.

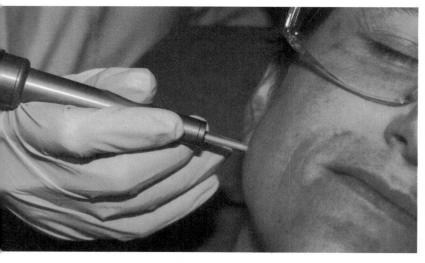

How does laser resurfacing work? Your dermatologist or plastic surgeon passes the laser over the target area of your skin and literally wipes off the layers of vaporized skin until he or she sees that a particular imperfection (wrinkle, spot) is less visible. This wiping away of dead skin forces your body to create brand-new layers of skin that are fresh and smooth. It takes about 7 to 10 days to grow new skin.

Deep facial lines will need a more intense laser workover to significantly reduce them, meaning additional passes of the laser over the face. Lighter wrinkles require only a quick pass to evaporate. As with every other procedure in cosmetic surgery, there are risks. With laser resurfacing, these include burns and changes in your skin color. It is important to have a trained, accredited doctor perform laser resurfacing (see page 190).

ask the experts

How long will the results of a laser resurfacing last?

A laser resurfacing (also called a **laser peel**) is generally a one-time procedure. However, if you have very deep lines or severe acne scarring, you may need a second treatment. And while the results are long lasting, they are not permanent. You are turning back the aging process, not stopping it. Wrinkles and lines will come back over time.

What is the best age to have laser treatment?

You need to be mature enough to deal with the post-operative discomfort and care. And you must be responsible enough to stay out of the sun for a time after treatment. Also, if you have acne and it isn't yet under control, laser resurfacing may not be advisable because you could get new acne scars.

I saw an ad for inexpensive laser leg-hair-removal treatments at a health spa. Is that safe?

Laser resurfacing for hair removal is becoming more and more popular. But unless it is done by a medical professional, it can be quite dangerous. In untrained hands, laser hair removal can result in burns and scarring. (For more on hair removal see page 78.)

CO₂ laser resurfacing

A high-tech treatment for fine and deep lines, and pigment problems

An alternative to chemical peels (see previous chapter) for skin resurfacing is the laser. The most common form of treatment involves a **CO₂** (carbon dioxide) laser to remove sun damage and signs of aging, such as wrinkles and fine lines (especially around the mouth and eyes), brown spots, uneven pigmentation, and some acne scars. Lasers can also be used to remove precancerous growths. A CO_2 laser is an **ablative laser**, which means it destroys the top layer of the skin.

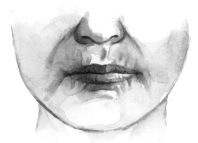

For the procedure, your doctor will start at the forehead and pass the laser over each area (eyes, each cheek, the nose, and around the mouth). He will wipe away layers of zapped skin until each imperfection is less visible. Some doctors will do one pass over the whole face and then come back for one or more additional passes; others will focus on one area at a time. The more passes done, the more aggressive the treatment. This typically one-time procedure takes about an hour.

Another ablative laser is the **erbium YAG**. It is usually tolerated a bit better than the CO_2 because less heat is transferred into the skin, resulting in less discomfort and less pinkness after treatment. Usually, just a topical anesthetic cream is used with the erbium laser, rather than mild sedation as with the CO_2. The erbium laser can also be used on the neck and chest, where the CO_2 would not be well tolerated. But it is not as effective as the CO_2 laser on deeper acne scars or lines.

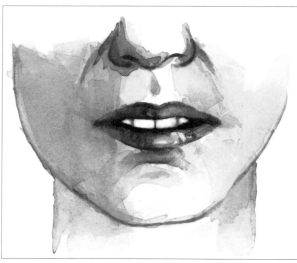

For those with fair skin, CO_2 laser resurfacing is effective at removing dense vertical wrinkles around the lips.

ask the experts

What are the risks involved with a CO_2 laser procedure?

Infection, scars, burns, prolonged redness, or the activation of a cold sore can occur with ablative lasers. The skin can also turn lighter or darker as it heals. If the skin darkens, it will fade, but it will take a long time to do so. If the skin turns lighter, it will be permanent. The erbium laser poses less risk of pigmentation changes than does the CO_2 laser. There is a higher risk of scarring when lasers are used on the neck and chest.

Should dark-skinned people undergo laser treatment?

Not CO_2 laser treatment. Darker-skinned people (Asian, African-American, Native American, Mediterranean) are at higher risk of having their skin turn darker or lighter as it heals. This is also true if you are very tanned. For info on treatment for darker-skinned people, see the next page.

What happens after laser surgery? What is recovery like?

You'll have a mask or dressing on your face and/or you'll have to soak your face several times a day for about a week. During that time you'll feel like you have a really bad sunburn. For the first week after the CO_2 laser procedure your skin will be red and raw, and you will have to apply ointment. At the end of the week your face will be pink, which should last from a few weeks to 6 months. It will take a week to 10 days before the crusting subsides and you're able to return to work. The neck and chest take longer to heal.

FEES

CO_2 Laser Resurfacing

Doctors' fees range from $2,000 to $7,000, depending on the extent of the area being treated and the type of laser being used. The erbium YAG laser treatment is around $1,000 less than the CO_2.

nonablative laser resurfacing

Laser treatment to soften lines, reduce acne scars, and for people of color

The best candidates for CO_2 laser resurfacing have fair, healthy, non-oily skin. For those who don't have time for prolonged healing, those who will not or cannot stay out of the sun (a requirement after CO_2 laser treatment), or those with darker skin there is **nonablative laser resurfacing**. This is the laser treatment for people of Mediterranean, Hispanic, Asian, African-American, or Indian descent, and for those who are deeply tanned, because the ablative CO_2 laser could leave the treated areas of their skin permanently lighter or darker.

The nonablative laser works by heating up the deeper layers of the skin while leaving the surface intact (unlike CO_2 and other ablative lasers, which leave the skin open and raw). The heat stimulates the formation of new collagen. The result? Softened lines, reduced acne scars, and improved texture. While this type of laser may not always reduce the number of lines on your face, it will seem to improve the quality of your skin. For deep wrinkles and creases, the only alternative may be a facelift (see page 176).

There are a number of nonablative laser systems, including the Photoderm, Cool Touch, and V-Beam. Five or six monthly sessions are necessary before you will see a difference. (A session can last from a few minutes to more than an hour, depending on the extent of the area being treated.) The trade-off between the nonablative and ablative (CO_2 and erbium YAG) lasers? With the nonablative you sacrifice some results for easier treatment and minimal recovery.

FEES

Nonablative Laser Resurfacing

Doctors' fees for a session can run from $300 to $1,000, depending on how much surface is being treated—a single area or the whole face.

ask the experts

What are the risks associated with nonablative laser procedures?

Unlike the fairly predictable outcome with ablative lasers, nonablative lasers have a more variable response. Your skin will be a little pink right after the procedure. And while recovery is minimal, as with ablative lasers, burns, scarring, infection, the activation of cold sores, and skin tone changes can occur.

CAUTIONARY TALE

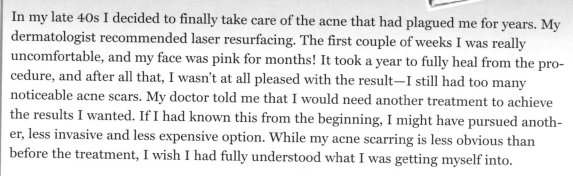

Lasering in on the facts

In my late 40s I decided to finally take care of the acne that had plagued me for years. My dermatologist recommended laser resurfacing. The first couple of weeks I was really uncomfortable, and my face was pink for months! It took a year to fully heal from the procedure, and after all that, I wasn't at all pleased with the result—I still had too many noticeable acne scars. My doctor told me that I would need another treatment to achieve the results I wanted. If I had known this from the beginning, I might have pursued another, less invasive and less expensive option. While my acne scarring is less obvious than before the treatment, I wish I had fully understood what I was getting myself into.

Jules M., Washington, D.C.

help for scars

Treatment to smooth and minimize scarring

While you can make a scar less obvious, no scar can be completely erased. Your dermatologist will need to evaluate your scar to determine the best course of treatment. If the scar is raised (**hypertrophic**), it can be flattened using topical steroid medications or injections, resurfacing (dermabrasion; see page 46), or surgery. Often, such scars improve on their own, though that can take a year or more. A depressed scar (**atrophic**) can be raised by injecting a soft-tissue filling material beneath it and/or by evening out the area with laser resurfacing.

If there is a difference in color, a red scar can be lightened with topical treatments or lasers, and a white scar can have tone added to it with **micropigmentation** (cosmetic tattooing; see page 64). Lasers can improve a difference in texture. If the scarred skin is pulled taut, restricting normal movement (as in two burned fingers less able to move independently after the healed skin forms a scar that knits them together), this **contracture** can be alleviated with surgery. A **keloid** (a thick, raised scar that grows beyond the area of the wound) is difficult to treat, whatever the method. For all scars, topical medications are typically used along with other treatments to achieve the best results.

ask the experts

What are the risks associated with these treatments?

You may have bleeding or infection. Your scar could return. Cortisone (steroid) injections can cause the skin to become too thin. If the steroid injected is too strong, it can thin out a scar so much that it will become a depression. And certain steroid or chemotherapeutic injections are not appropriate for children or pregnant women.

I have a large scarred area from an accident. Is there another option for me?

For larger scars or those that don't respond to less invasive forms of treatment there are skin grafts and flap surgery. These complex surgical procedures usually require general anesthesia in a hospital setting. You will have two surgical sites—the area your healthy skin is taken from and the scar area it is transferred to—so recovery can last several weeks or months. You may need to wear a compression garment for as long as 12 months.

What about the results?

While no scar can be removed completely, it can be greatly improved. The degree of change depends primarily on the scar's size, elevation, and texture, as well as the quality of your skin. If you treat a scar surgically and it actually seems worse at first, don't panic—it may take at least a year before the final results become apparent.

Do the scars on my face need to be treated differently from those on my body?

Facial scars differ from those on the rest of the body in that they allow you more treatment options. For example, the CO_2 laser, which is fine for the face, is not appropriate for the body. The same is true for dermabrasion, which can soften facial scars. Also unique to the face are **Botox** injections (see page 34), which can temporarily decrease the appearance of scars on the forehead and crow's feet areas, in the same way they're used to treat wrinkles.

FEES

Scar Revision

Doctors' fees vary as much as the variety of treatments. But you must have the treatment that is appropriate for your scar, so shopping for a bargain isn't the answer. Full-face laser resurfacing costs between $4,000 and $6,000. For a scar that needs to be injected with collagen, one injection is roughly $350 to $500. A scar that needs to be injected with cortisone or a chemotherapeutic agent costs about $150 per treatment, depending on its size. These are all multiple-treatment processes. While these elective procedures aren't typically covered by insurance, if your scar revision is necessary because of an accident or to improve function, it may be covered, at least in part.

tattoo removal

How to lose that artistic statement

Tired of literally wearing your heart on your sleeve? Or have you developed an allergy to your tattoo (which can happen years later)? Tattoo removal is possible, but not easy. Before lasers, your doctor would only be able to cut out a tattoo or use **dermabrasion** (see page 46) to sand down the skin, but both methods can leave a large white scar where the tattoo was.

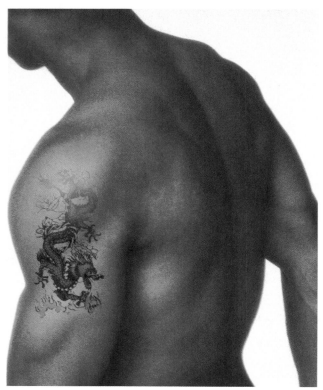

Today there are a few lasers suited to tattoo removal, but some tattoos will respond better than others. The laser's energy breaks the ink pigment into small granules that the body's systems can remove naturally. The success of the treatment depends on how deep the pigment is in the skin, the type of ink used, and the tattoo's location, size, and how long it has been on the skin.

The process can require 4 to 12 treatments, using local anesthesia. Unfortunately, thanks to newer inks that are especially hard to remove, the tattoo often cannot be eliminated 100%. Instead, the tattoo area may be lighter than your normal skin tone.

ask the experts

What are the risks associated with tattoo removal?

The biggest risks are scarring and incomplete removal. Some pigments used in tattoos, especially on the face, turn black when they are treated with a laser. That blackened tattoo typically does not respond to other lasers and will need to be surgically removed, which will leave a scar. (This is common with the removal of lip lining tattoos, called **micropigmentation**; see the next page for more on this.) Other complications include infection, change of pigmentation, and change of texture.

What does recovery involve?

You will typically experience crusting. The scabbing will take about 2 weeks to heal.

Can lasers remove tattoos I got from radiation therapy?

Radiation for cancer treatment sometimes involves marking the skin with tattoos to help target the beams to the tumors. With a few treatments, lasers can remove or at least significantly lighten these tattoos.

FEES

Tattoo Removal

Costs for tattoo removal vary with the size of the tattoo and where it is on the body. In some big tattoo practices, a nurse may do the treatment, which may be less expensive than the doctor's rates. It will run several hundred dollars per treatment.

permanent makeup

Cosmetic tattooing can enhance your features

You may want to have tattooing for cosmetic reasons. **Micropigmentation** is the (relatively) permanent application, or tattooing, of makeup. It is most commonly done for eyeliner, lip liner, and eyebrows, though some have eye shadow or blush tattooed on. It can be extremely useful for those who have suffered the loss of facial hair or have discoloration or scarring due to cancer or some other trauma.

While aestheticians are licensed in many states to apply permanent makeup, for your safety it is best done by a trained medical professional (unless your dermatologist can refer you to an aesthetician who specializes in micropigmentation).

Here's how it works: A numbing cream (or an injection if the treatment involves the lips) is applied to the area first. (You may be sent to a physician or dentist to have the mouth injected to numb it.) Then the needles with pigment are applied. The procedure is usually done in small increments, and spread over several treatments. Each session lasts a half hour to 2 hours, depending on how large an area is being treated and how many areas there are. The treated area may scab for about a week. While referred to as permanent, this tattooing will fade over three to five years, so expect to have to touch it up over time.

FEES

Micropigmentation

Fees vary significantly depending on the training of the person performing the technique and the number of areas being treated, but typically run from several hundred dollars to $1,000 per treatment.

ask the experts

What is the most important consideration with micropigmentation?

Your key consideration is the practitioner. Look for someone with extensive experience not in regular tattoo application but in this specialty, which requires precision in tattooing very fine lines and tiny dots to create natural-looking, lip- and skin-color-matching makeup. You want someone who can subtly enhance color to deal with fading edges, scars that have turned white, or white spots, in order to blend them into the surrounding skin.

What are the risks with micropigmentation?

There is a risk of having an allergic reaction to the dye. A lip tattoo could trigger a herpes outbreak (cold sores). And any tattoo could result in hepatitis if the equipment used is not sterile. Also, the pigments used in tattoos are not FDA regulated.

now what do I do?

Answers to common questions

Should I avoid sun exposure after a cosmetic skin procedure?

Many of the skin-smoothing techniques uncover fresh layers of skin that should not be exposed to the sun as they heal, so always use sunblock and wear a wide-brimmed hat. (See page 30 for more on this.) If you have resurfacing done around the eyes, wear sunglasses that have 100% filters for UVA and UVB rays.

Can techniques be combined to treat different problem areas?

Yes, most of the treatments let you mix and match types of procedures. Your doctor should select the appropriate method for each area and problem you want to address.

Should I have a facelift before I do any skin resurfacing?

The facelift and laser resurfacing are complementary procedures. Skin resurfacing can seem to give you a mini-facelift, but it won't fix sagging skin, which needs to be cut away with a facelift. It's not uncommon to have a facelift followed by a skin-smoothing or resurfacing treatment to address crow's feet and other lines not remedied by a facelift. (For more on the facelift, see page 176.)

What can I do for the very noticeable blood vessels on my face?

Rosacea (an adult acne), sun damage, and genetics are the most common causes of blood vessel problems on the face. Treatment typically requires 3 to 5 laser sessions done a month apart, to allow the blood vessels to become relatively stable so that your doctor can see what needs to be treated next. Sometimes doctors will combine laser treatment with **sclerotherapy**—some injections on the cheeks—depending on how large the blood vessels are. (See page 150 for more on this.)

Can lasers remove my stretch marks?

Lasers can remove the pink or redness of stretch marks as well as improve the quality and texture of your skin. It will require several treatments to achieve the desired result.

What are Photofacials?

These are procedures done with the nonablative Photoderm laser to improve the effects of facial **photo-aging** (sun damage resulting in highly visible blood vessels and brown spots). Multiple treatments are necessary. Along with improvement of your appearance, studies have shown that the use of this laser results in some production of new collagen. A session is roughly $500 to $1,000. While there is minimal recovery, you could experience pain, bruising, scabbing, or scarring, and the skin can turn lighter or darker.

now where do I go?!

CONTACTS

American Academy of Dermatology
www.aad.org
888-462-DERM

American Society for
Dermatologic Surgery
www.asds-net.org
800-441-ASDS

American Society of Plastic Surgeons
www.plasticsurgery.org
847-228-9900

American Society for
Aesthetic Plastic Surgery
www.surgery.org
212-921-0500

American Academy of Facial Plastic
and Reconstructive Surgery
www.aafprs.org
800-332-FACE

ADDITIONAL INFORMATION

U.S. Food and Drug Administration
www.fda.gov

Cosmetic Surgery News
www.cosmeticsurgery-news.com

Cosmetic Surgery & Skin Care News
www.cosmetic-surgery-news.com

Chapter 4

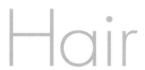

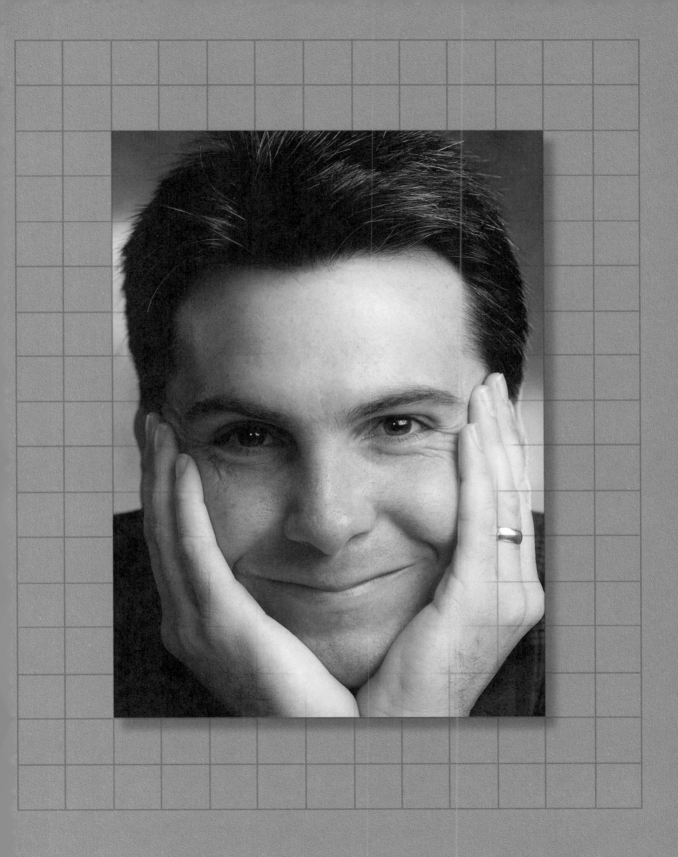

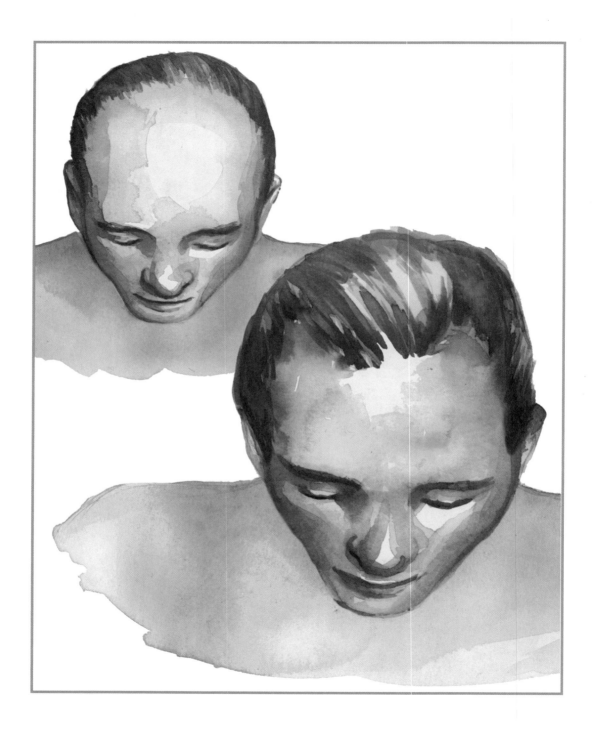

What Mother Nature takes away, a plastic surgeon will endeavor to give back. Perhaps nowhere is this more evident than with a hair transplant. Here, a doctor can take strands of your own hair that are genetically hardy and graft them onto bald spots to create a fuller, more youthful head of hair.

baldness explained

Blame it on your parents

If it's any comfort, two out of every three men and one out of every five women will experience some kind of hair loss or baldness. This slow, tormenting process is termed **pattern baldness**. (Its medical name is **androgenetic alopecia**.)

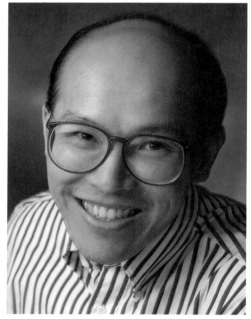

Male balding often leaves just a fringe of hearty hair around the head. Plastic surgeons can transplant some of this hair to fill out balding areas.

What causes typical pattern baldness? A combination of hormonal activity and heredity, which together produce thinning hair and pattern changes. This genetic double-whammy accounts for 95% of hair loss. (Less common causes include illness, certain medications, and even, some say, extreme stress.)

Male pattern baldness usually begins with a receding hairline along with fallout or thinning at the crown. This generally progresses over a lifetime, and may leave only a horseshoe-shaped fringe around the sides and back of the head. Female pattern baldness—typically due to hormonal changes, particularly in menopause—usually consists of thinning over the entire scalp with the front rim usually preserved.

The age at which thinning begins and your family history of baldness are significant factors in predicting how much loss you will experience. What are your chances of losing your hair? Since it's a genetic predisposition, take a look at your family. For men, hair loss is usually passed down from your father and/or your mother's father; for women, it's typically a pattern from your mother.

ask the experts

What is DHT?

It is the real culprit behind hair loss. **DHT**, or **dihydrotestos-terone**, is the byproduct of the male hormone **androgen**. DHT binds to hair **follicles** (roots) and shrinks them over time.

How do the medicines Rogaine and Propecia restore hair?

Both these prescription medicines combat hair loss. Rogaine (**minoxidil**) is a topical treatment that can prevent further hair loss and regrow hair, though how much is a great source of debate—and once you stop using it the regrown hair may fall out. Propecia (**finasteride**) is a pill that will maintain your current hair count and generate some hair growth. It is not effective for women, especially after menopause. Both medicines stop working the minute you stop taking them. Yes, that's right, you need to take them for the rest of your life, or hair loss ensues. These drugs should not be taken by women who plan to have children because their effects on a developing fetus are unknown.

hair transplants

How to artfully transfer hair to bald spots

Not all hairs on the scalp are created equal. Some are genetically coded to fall out, others to remain and grow. Almost everyone has a horseshoe-shaped fringe of hair (going from ear to ear) that is genetically programmed always to grow. The good news is that hairs from this area of **donor dominance** can be removed and transplanted to balding areas on the head (and elsewhere on the body), where they will take root and grow. This procedure doesn't create any new hair; rather, it redistributes hair more aesthetically to cover bald spots.

A hair transplant is done using local anesthesia. The surgeon cuts out hair follicles (taking the skin in which they reside) from the back or sides of your head and closes up the scalp. Next, the surgeon or his technicians cut up the removed portion of scalp into individual **grafts** (pieces of hair-bearing skin), each containing 1 or 2 hairs (**micrografts**), 3 to 4 hairs (**minigrafts**), or 7 to 15 hairs (**plugs**). The surgeon then makes little holes in the balding scalp areas into which he'll deposit the grafts. To achieve a more natural and fuller appearance he'll attempt to position the hairs so they all grow in the same direction as the existing hairs, and are well spaced. The goal for someone with significant balding is not to create a really thick head of hair, it's to frame the face so that when you look at the person you see a mature man with thinning hair. With minimal balding you can create a thicker looking head of hair.

A session generally takes 2 to 6 hours to transplant anywhere from 400 to 700 grafts. Follow-up sessions are done in 3 to 12 months, depending on the cycle of hair growth and rest, and healing time. The entire process can take as long as two years. Some people opt for **megasessions**, in which 1,000 to 2,000 grafts are done at one time. While this shortens the process, it's a more involved operation, lasting about 6 hours. And the price is significantly higher.

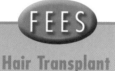

FEES

Hair Transplant

This procedure is typically priced by the graft, which is a group of one to four hairs. For multiple sessions over a 1- to 2-year period, the surgeon's fees can range from $3,000 to $9,000. The megasession process can cost as much as $15,000. A hair transplant is covered by insurance only if it is necessary due to burns, or another injury or accident to the scalp.

ask the experts

What risks are associated with this procedure?

You will have scarring at the spot from which you're removing hair, but it should be hidden. Subsequent hair loss may give you the appearance of having patches of hair where the initial grafts were placed, requiring additional surgery to correct this unnatural look. Hair color, texture, and waviness may affect the final result.

What considerations are there for women?

Men almost always have a sufficient fringe of dominant hair for transplanting, but women tend to have more thinning than receding. Their fringe hair is often insufficient to use in thickening up hair that's thin all over. In such cases, a wig might be the only effective solution, though medication offers some hope (see page 73).

What is recovery like?

There will be some discomfort, and for a day or two you'll have a dressing covering your scalp to keep the grafts in position. You may have some swelling around the forehead and upper eyelids. After 48 hours you'll be able to use a baby shampoo. Scabs will form and take a week to fall off. You can return to work in 1 week, but avoid strenuous activity for 2 weeks. For up to 3 months you may experience some numbness in the areas the hair was transplanted from and to.

How long will the results last?

You can expect to see about a half-inch of new hair growth per month. The survival rate for transplanted hair is around 95%, so if you move 100 hairs, 95 of them should live—and last a lifetime in their new area (though this is not always predictable).

scalp reduction

Cutting out the bald spot

While hair transplants can be cosmetically very helpful, the thickness or density of such hair will never be as much as the normal scalp. If you want really thick hair, or if you have too much of a balding area to adequately cover with transplants alone, you may opt for **scalp reduction surgery**. This procedure involves taking the part of the scalp that has thick hair and stretching it a bit, then cutting out the bald spot and replacing it with part of that expanded hairy area. The best candidate for scalp reduction surgery is a man whose hair loss has stopped.

Scalp reduction requires several surgeries because there is a limit to how much of the scalp can be removed at any one time. The amount decreases with each successive operation. During the first procedure, your surgeon will cut out close to two inches of scalp and sew the remaining parts back together. In the second, he will remove about one inch. The third will remove less than an inch. Generally, each surgery takes 1 to 2 hours and is performed under general anesthesia.

To achieve optimum results, you can combine scalp reduction with **hair transplants** (see the previous page). Because the reduction surgery will decrease the area that will need to be seeded by the transplants, it will be easier to achieve the look of a full head of hair. And the transplants will both cover up the scars from the scalp reduction procedure and thicken other areas of the scalp.

The results should be permanent, but the scalp, like other skin, can stretch back and undo what you gained from the procedure. If this occurs, not only will your baldness start to return, but **stretch-back scarring**, in which tension causes the scars to widen and become more visible, can occur.

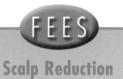

FEES

Scalp Reduction

Fees range from $1,000 to $4,000, depending on the extent of your balding. Because the results are best when this operation is done along with hair transplants, you might want to include that price when calculating your total payout. The final expense can be anywhere from $10,000 to $20,000.

ask the experts

What risks are associated with this procedure?

Scarring and infection can occur, but the worst complication is **slot deformity**. Men typically have a bald area in the middle of the head, from front to back. It is this area that is cut out and pulled together in the center. The hair that was growing on the sides of the head is now in the center, but will continue to grow in its natural pattern, possibly leaving you with a slot, or groove, in the middle of your head. Combining scalp reduction with hair transplants can camouflage this problem.

What is recovery like?

After surgery, you may have pain and swelling for a few days, and your scalp will feel achy and tight. You can return to work in about a week, but no strenuous activity for up to 3 weeks. It can take a year or more to see the final results.

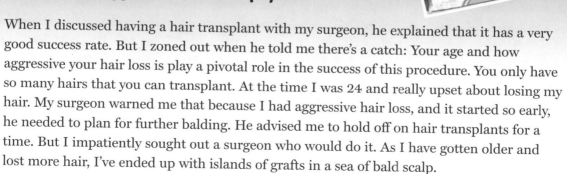

CAUTIONARY TALE

When being aggressive doesn't pay off

When I discussed having a hair transplant with my surgeon, he explained that it has a very good success rate. But I zoned out when he told me there's a catch: Your age and how aggressive your hair loss is play a pivotal role in the success of this procedure. You only have so many hairs that you can transplant. At the time I was 24 and really upset about losing my hair. My surgeon warned me that because I had aggressive hair loss, and it started so early, he needed to plan for further balding. He advised me to hold off on hair transplants for a time. But I impatiently sought out a surgeon who would do it. As I have gotten older and lost more hair, I've ended up with islands of grafts in a sea of bald scalp.

Jessie P., Chappaqua, New York

removing unwanted hair

Should you choose a laser or electrolysis?

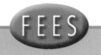

FEES

Hair Removal

Laser hair removal costs around $400 to $500 per treatment—and you'll need 3 to 4 sessions on average, depending on the body part you want treated. A large area, such as the back, can cost between $800 and $1,500 because it takes longer to do. Electrolysis runs from $50 to $150 for a 1-hour treatment, depending on the amount and thickness of the hair being removed. Electrolysis requires many hours of treatment over the course of several weeks or months. With either procedure, be sure to take the multiple sessions into account when you're calculating your costs.

Hair often grows where it is not wanted. Happily, there are two major nonsurgical ways to permanently remove hair: **electrolysis** and **laser treatment**. With electrolysis, a wire or probe is inserted into each hair **follicle** (root) to deliver a low electric current that destroys it. Laser hair removal uses a beam of low energy that, when absorbed by the pigment in the hair follicle, permanently disables that follicle.

Both are safe, effective, and relatively painless. Both require multiple treatments to complete the task, though the individual sessions are fairly quick—anywhere from a few minutes to an hour. However, there are trade-offs associated with each method. Electrolysis is a far more painstaking and prolonged process because each hair is treated individually, unlike a laser, which removes more than one hair at a time. On the other hand, laser hair removal, while far quicker, is less thorough. While electrolysis can eliminate every hair, the laser process will leave behind a few fine hairs.

Laser hair removal is the method of choice when it comes to treating large areas such as a man's back or chest. With a laser, a man's back can be treated in an hour. Laser removal is also ideal for a woman's underarms, legs, and face—the upper lip can be done in only three minutes—providing you're willing to have some hairs left, which could then be removed with electrolysis.

ask the experts

What risks are associated with these procedures?

You may experience some discomfort while undergoing electrolysis or laser hair removal. The laser may cause some redness, blistering, and temporary skin discoloration. In rare instances, scarring may occur with laser treatment.

Why do I have to pace my laser procedures?

The laser can only pick up hairs that are present, not those that are in a resting phase, which all hairs go through every few weeks. This alone will require you to go for a minimum of 3 to 4 treatments every 4 to 6 weeks, depending on the body part you're treating. And while you will enjoy a very good reduction of hair, there will always be some hair that seems not to respond. In particular, a laser will not work on light-colored hair, such as silver, white, and even some shades of blonde, because it can't pick up light colors. Also, because a person's hair must be darker than their skin for laser hair removal to work, people of color may not be good candidates for laser treatment. Even tanned people with dark hair must wait for their tan to fade before undergoing this process.

What is recovery like and how long will the results last?

Recovery from both treatments is immediate. The results from a single session are permanent, but incomplete—both methods require multiple sessions to clear a body part of most or all hair. While you might have 3 to 4 months of no hair growth following a laser treatment, long-term there will always be a few hairs remaining, so your days of waxing, plucking, or having electrolysis aren't necessarily over.

now what do I do?

Answers to common questions

I heard that shortly after a hair transplant some of my new hair will fall out! Is this true?

Don't be alarmed—it's normal for your new hair to fall out in the 2 to 6 weeks following a transplant. This happens when the hairs go into a resting phase, part of their natural life cycle. In about 3 to 6 months the hairs will start to grow again and will continue to do so for about a year. That's when you will see the final results of your transplant.

Are there special considerations for African-Americans when doing hair transplantation surgery?

African-Americans tend to have lower hair density in the donor area (the fringe of hair at the back of the head from which the hair is transplanted), which could make hair transplantation impractical. On the other hand, the characteristic curl of the hair can make up for having fewer hairs because it gives an impression of density. And keloids—large, irregularly shaped scars—occur more frequently among people with darker skin.

Are there other factors, besides heredity, that cause hair loss, and can I do anything to prevent or reduce it?

Thyroid irregularities, the use of certain medications, and even poor diet can contribute to hair loss. Hormonal changes in women, such as those brought about by birth control pills or menopause, can also cause this problem. Women may also experience temporary hair loss following childbirth.

Can hair be transplanted from any part of the body to the scalp?

Hair from the back and chest can be transplanted to the scalp, but since it has a different texture, it may look unnatural on your head.

I've lost my eyebrows to an injury. What can I do about it?

If you've lost your eyelashes or eyebrows to disease or injury, or simply want to enhance their appearance, consider hair transplantation. With this technique, you can move hairs from the back of your head to another part of your body. You can create eyelashes, a mustache, a beard, even pubic hair. You can make a close match by taking finer hair from your head for, say, eyebrows. But it won't look exactly like eyebrow hair because the grafted hair will continue to grow the same way the hair on your head grows, so you will need to trim it and possibly flatten it with gel or wax.

Now where do I go?!

CONTACTS

International Society of Hair
Restoration Surgery
www.ishrs.org
800-444-2737

American Hair Loss Council
www.ahlc.org
888-873-9719

American Society of Plastic Surgeons
www.plasticsurgery.org
847-228-9900

ADDITIONAL INFORMATION

**Hair Savers for Women:
A Complete Guide to Preventing
and Treating Hair Loss**
By Maggie Greenwood-Robinson

**The Everyman's Guide to Hair
Replacement**
By Dr. Richard Fleming

Cosmetic Surgery News
www.cosmeticsurgery-news.com

Chapter 5

The Nose

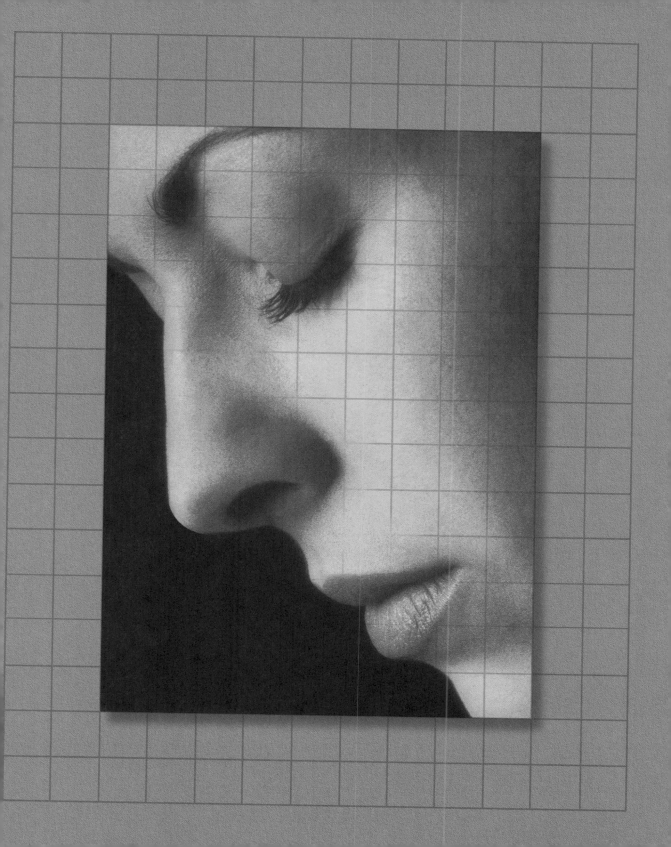

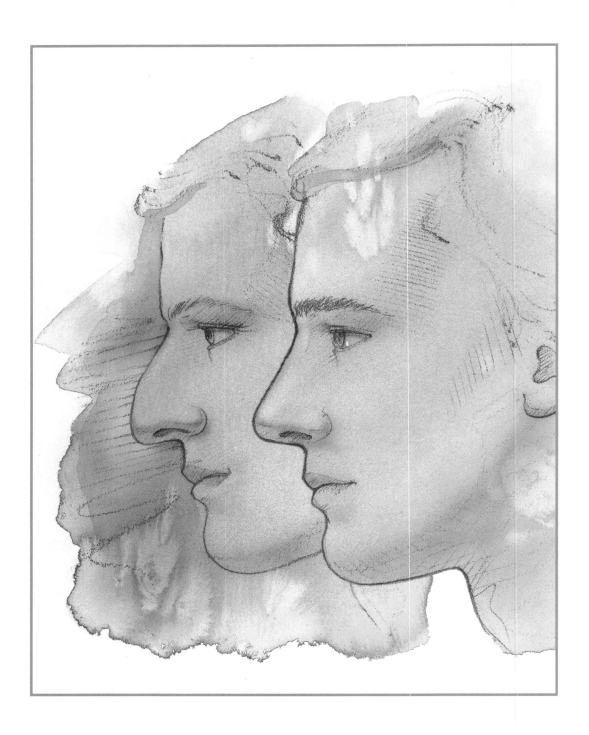

The face is a wonderful blend of features. When one is out of balance, the whole face suffers. Often the culprit is the nose. Whether it's a reduction, enlargement, or other work called for on the nose, cosmetic surgery can create or restore proportion and symmetry.

the basic nose job

Reducing a bumpy or bulbous nose

The aesthetic surgical reshaping of the nose is called **rhinoplasty,** and it's among the top five cosmetic surgery procedures performed each year. Your nose is composed of three layers: an inner lining, bone and cartilage, and outer skin. To make the bridge narrower, your surgeon will make an incision on the inside of each nostril (to avoid visible scarring). He is then able to reshape the nose by altering the cartilage and bone.

A bump may be fixed by carving out excess cartilage and bone. In some cases, your doctor may have to break the bones so that they can be repositioned. A bulbous or droopy tip can be reduced by removing some of the cartilage or by suturing (stitching) the cartilage to bend it into a more pleasing shape. Too-wide nostrils can be narrowed by removing one or two small wedges of skin at the base of the nostrils, where they join the upper lip. The tiny scars that result should be camouflaged by the natural crease there.

Reduction surgery for the bridge or tip of your nose or your nostrils takes roughly 30 minutes for each area. The procedure can be performed using local or general anesthesia.

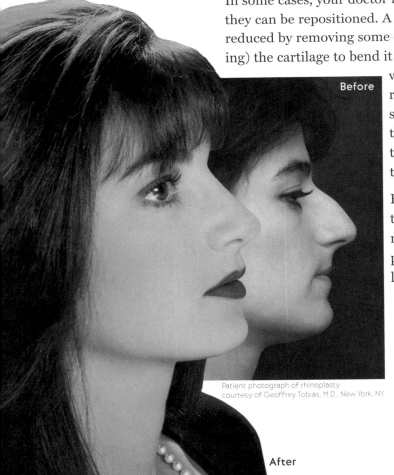

Before

Patient photograph of rhinoplasty
courtesy of Geoffrey Tobias, M.D., New York, NY

After

ask the experts

What happens after the surgery? What is recovery like?

The bridge of your nose will be black and blue, and swollen for a number of days. Your nose will be taped, and for about 5 days you'll have to wear a splint or cast on it for protection and to help maintain its new shape. A mustache-like dressing under your nose and/or gauze packing in your nostrils may have to remain in place for one to several days. You must not blow your nose for about a week. It will be about a month before you can resume strenuous physical activity, and you must avoid hitting your nose or getting it sunburned for up to 8 weeks.

How long will the results last?

Reductive rhinoplasty is permanent—except as aging takes its normal toll. You might notice a minor imperfection such as a very small bump as the bones and tissue heal. This can occur from the formation of scar tissue, calcium deposits, or the shifting of bone or tissue over time. Another procedure six months to a year later, after the swelling has completely subsided, can correct this.

What should my expectations be for my new nose?

You can't just point to a picture of a nose in a magazine and expect your surgeon to give you that nose. Your doctor must work within the limitations of your anatomy and the inherent characteristics of your skin, bone, and cartilage to achieve your new look.

What are the risks associated with this procedure?

Scar tissue from the incisions could cause breathing problems. Also, at the outset, you may experience the sensation of having difficulty breathing as you adjust to your smaller nose.

FEES

Nose Reduction

Surgeons' fees for work on the bridge, tip and/or nostrils range from $2,500 to $6,500, depending on the extent of the work done.

enhancing the nose

Building a better bridge, leaving a good tip

Augmentation rhinoplasty is the procedure used to build up the bridge of the nose or to reshape the tip to create a stronger profile. For the surgery, your doctor can use synthetic material, such as solid silicone or Gortex, or tissue taken from elsewhere in your body—usually cartilage from the **septum** (the thin dividing membrane in your nose), behind the ear, or a rib. Bone, most often transplanted from the hip, can also be used. If cartilage or bone is to be transplanted from another part of the body, it's removed during a separate procedure that is done at the same time.

Your surgeon will carve the bone, cartilage or synthetic material to create the proper curves and angles to enhance the shape of the bridge. It is then layered over the bone or cartilage within the nose. The edges of the new material must be very thin and tapered so that it blends in with the surrounding tissue. The skin holds it in place.

For the tip, a fair amount of sculpted cartilage, grafts are necessary to achieve the desired effect. It takes about 30 minutes for either single surgery; an hour or so if a transplant is involved. The procedures can be done at an outpatient facility or hospital, using local or general anesthesia.

ask the experts

What would make me a poor candidate for this procedure?

If the skin on your nose, especially the tip, is very thick and inflexible, it will be difficult to effectively change the shape of your nose. This complication worsens as we age and the skin becomes increasingly less elastic.

What are the risks associated with this procedure?

There is a slight risk of infection. Your body could reject the synthetic material. Small blood vessels in your nose could burst, causing very small but permanent red spots. Additional surgery may be required to correct distortion in the shape, which can occur over time, or to smooth out ridges that show as you age.

What is recovery like?

Recovery is similar to that of reduction rhinoplasty (see page 87). As for any rhinoplasty, it can take as long as 12 to 18 months for all evidence of swelling to disappear. This is especially true for the procedure to reshape the tip by adding layers of cartilage. It should also be noted that women tend to have slightly thinner skin than men, so they will be more likely to notice small imperfections after surgery.

How long will the results last?

While the results should be permanent, your nose will show the natural signs of aging over time.

FEES

Augmentation Rhinoplasty

Surgeons' fees can range from $3,000 to $6,500. Add another 20% if you're having cartilage or bone taken from the ear, rib, or hip.

fixing a broken nose

Treatment for the traumatized nose

Your nose is under attack! It's sneezed through, blown, exposed to sun, cold and wind, and bumped without much notice—until something goes wrong. When bad things happen to good noses, doctors can perform one of two procedures to fix the problem.

Revision (or secondary) **rhinoplasty** is used to correct a previous surgery. You'll have to wait six months to a year after the original surgery to redo your nose. The wait is necessary to allow the swelling to disappear completely. **Traumatic rhinoplasty** is surgery to treat a broken or damaged nose. Both can be done in an outpatient facility or a hospital, using local or general anesthesia.

Like augmentation surgery (see page 88), revision rhinoplasty requires a cartilage or bone graft or the use of synthetic material to rebuild the bridge or tip. The surgical techniques are similar. However, there are complications associated with the revision procedure. For example, scar tissue from the original procedure may force the surgeon to make external incisions, which leave visible scarring. Fortunately, scars can be smoothed out or camouflaged through **dermabrasion** (a kind of surgical sandpapering of the skin; for more on this procedure see page 46). Revision surgery lasts from $1^1/_2$ to $2^1/_2$ hours.

With traumatic rhinoplasty, a fracture that has set generally has to be rebroken and repositioned. Also, tissue that may have collapsed from injury would have to be built back up, again, with techniques used in augmentation surgery. This procedure takes from 1 to 2 hours.

FEES

Revision and Traumatic Rhinoplasties

Surgeons' fees for revision rhinoplasty are slightly higher than for primary rhinoplasty, ranging from $4,000 to $7,000. This procedure may be partially covered by insurance if there is internal scarring or tissue collapse that is causing breathing problems. Fees for traumatic rhinoplasty range from $3,000 to $6,500. Some portion may be covered by insurance, depending on the underlying cause.

@sk the experts

What are the risks associated with these procedures?

Possible physical complications following either procedure include infection, bleeding, and breathing problems. Revision rhinoplasty can also pose psychological challenges at the outset because the patient may have been traumatized by the disappointing outcome of the original surgery.

What is recovery like?

Recovery is the same as for reductive rhinoplasty (see page 86). In addition, you may experience headaches, some bleeding, and congestion.

CAUTIONARY TALE

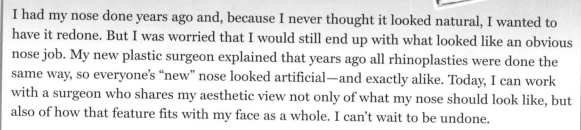

The un-nose job

I had my nose done years ago and, because I never thought it looked natural, I wanted to have it redone. But I was worried that I would still end up with what looked like an obvious nose job. My new plastic surgeon explained that years ago all rhinoplasties were done the same way, so everyone's "new" nose looked artificial—and exactly alike. Today, I can work with a surgeon who shares my aesthetic view not only of what my nose should look like, but also of how that feature fits with my face as a whole. I can't wait to be undone.

Liz S., Philadelphia, Pennsylvania

breathing problems?

Addressing the deviated septum

FEES

Deviated Septum

Surgeons' fees range from $1,000 to $3,500. The procedure is usually covered by insurance if you can demonstrate a history of breathing or sinus problems (infections and headaches) that have not responded to nonsurgical treatment.

A **deviated septum** is a medical condition in which a blockage in the nasal passages can cause difficulty breathing or recurring sinus infections. While the surgery to correct it, **septoplasty**, is commonly done in conjunction with rhinoplasty (the reshaping of the appearance of the nose), it is not a cosmetic treatment. The combined procedure is called **septorhinoplasty**.

The septum, which is mostly flexible cartilage, is the natural partition that divides the two air passages and extends from the nostrils to deep into the nasal cavity all the way to the throat. Normally the septum is relatively smooth and flat, but when it's deviated it has jagged folds that can block airflow through the nose. To correct this, your surgeon will make a single incision within the nostril and stretch out the septum, or he will remove its jagged folds to make it smooth. Because he is not slicing the nose open there are no external incisions, so no scars will be visible. The surgery takes 30 minutes, using local or general anesthesia. It can be done in an outpatient facility or a hospital.

While septoplasty should reasonably improve your breathing, it's not a cure for all breathing problems.

ask the experts

What risks are associated with this procedure?

Scar tissue may form between the septum and the lining of the nasal cavity, which can cause a recurrence or even a worsening of the nasal obstruction. You could end up with a perforation (hole) in the septum, which could cause more breathing difficulties or make your nose whistle when you breathe through it. Mucus may build up within the perforation and create a new blockage. This hole may be permanent if it is too large and difficult to repair. If the septum heals improperly or you sustain an injury to your nose, the deviation could recur. Should this happen, you can have the surgery redone after waiting a few months to allow the swelling to subside.

What is recovery like?

You will have a small mustache-like dressing under your nose along with a splint supporting the outside of your nose. While you will be able to breathe through your nose a little, for the first few days you'll mostly have to breathe through your mouth. Expect to have a stuffy nose, off and on, for a few weeks. Within a week after surgery, your doctor will use a cotton swab and/or a thin suction tube to gently clean out your nose and open the nasal passageways. You can resume strenuous activity after a month.

What would make me a poor candidate for this surgery?

If you have certain medical conditions that affect your ability to control bleeding, such as hemophilia or significant high blood pressure, or if you use anticoagulants (such as aspirin, the herbal remedy ginkgo, or medication due to a stroke), this surgery may not be suitable for you.

now what do I do?

Answers to common questions

How can I tell what I might look like if I have my nose done?

Have your surgeon show you "before" and "after" photos of people who had problems similar to yours. While computer imaging can be helpful, it can give a false representation of how you will heal. A better, low-tech approach is to blow up "before" pictures of your nose, taken from various angles, and review them with your surgeon, clearly pointing out and discussing your areas of concern.

What if I'm not really sure if my nose is too big or something else is out of balance with my face?

Rhinoplasty alone will not give you the desired effect if your other features are out of proportion. For example, your nose may appear to be oversized when, in fact, you have a weak chin. Look in a three-way mirror and closely examine your profile. Then discuss your options with a plastic surgeon. Other plastic surgery procedures, such as **chin augmentation** (implants; see page 170) and jaw restructuring (see page 110) are commonly done together with rhinoplasty.

What age is too young to have nose surgery? Is any age too old?

Children shouldn't have surgery until after their noses are fully developed—age 14 for girls and 15 or 16 for boys. If you don't have any medical conditions that may complicate the surgery (such as high blood pressure, or clotting problems), there is no such thing as being too old to have a nose job.

Can I wear my glasses after nose surgery?

You may have to stop wearing glasses for the first few days or weeks following surgery. If that is not an option, your surgeon can instruct you on how to use tape or another device to support them so that they will not place any stress on your nose.

What happens if I have a nosebleed after nose surgery?

For up to 3 weeks following any type of nose surgery, it's common to experience nosebleeds. These can last up to 30 minutes and typically stop on their own. Avoid activities that raise blood pressure and could bring on a serious nosebleed, including blowing your nose hard, bending over, and strenuous activity (including sex), for a week or so. Also, try not to become constipated, since straining can also cause a severe post-operative nosebleed. See your doctor if the bleeding persists.

Should I tell my other healthcare providers that I've had a nose job?

Always tell your medical practitioners when you've had any form of surgery, whether it was done in a hospital, and what type of anesthesia (general or local) was used. That way they have a complete medical history to provide you with the best care.

Now where do I go?!

CONTACTS	
American Society of Plastic Surgeons **www.plasticsurgery.org** 888-475-2784	American Academy of Facial Plastic and Reconstructive Surgery **www.aafprs.org** 800-332-FACE
American Society for Aesthetic Plastic Surgery **www.surgery.org** 888-272-7711	**ADDITIONAL INFORMATION** Cosmetic Surgery News **www.cosmeticsurgery-news.com**

Chapter 6

Lighten Up

Contour a New Look

Bonding

Cosmetic Dentistry

Veneers

Braces for Grown-ups

Jaw Restructuring

Now What Do I Do?

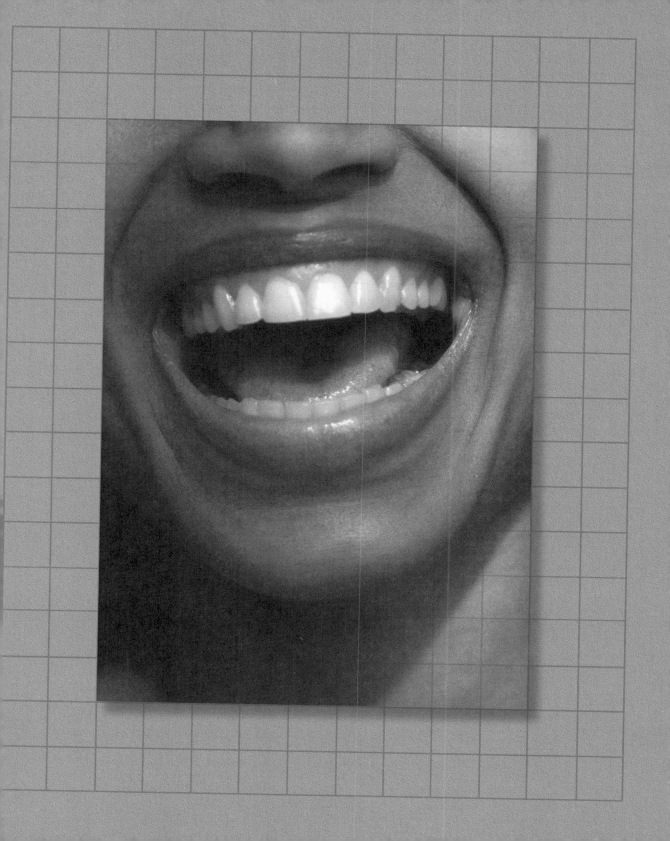

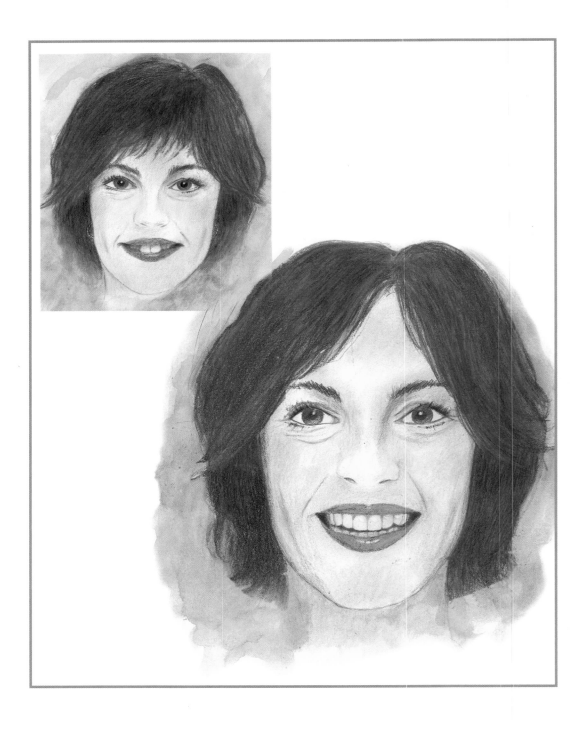

The smile says it all. Straight, well-formed, bright teeth do wonders to boost the conversation, while crooked, stained, chipped, or bucked teeth can steal attention away from your words. Cosmetic dental and orthodontia work can fix just about any tooth- or jaw-related appearance problem.

lighten up

Bleaching can turn up the wattage in your smile

If your teeth are less than pearly white, there is help. You can have your teeth bleached, either at your dentist's office or at home. The at-home system, done under your dentist's supervision, is the most popular—and most reliable—method for whitening moderately stained or discolored teeth. Here's how it works: Your dentist takes an impression of your teeth, from which he'll make a plaster model to shape a custom-fitted, plastic mouth tray (like a mouth guard) for home use.

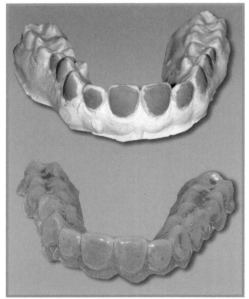

From a plaster model of your teeth, your dentist can create a plastic mouth tray in which you pour a bit of bleaching gel. You then wear the mouth tray for a specified time.

At home you'll fill the tray with a bleaching gel (10%, 16%, or 22% carbamide peroxide, which your dentist will prescribe) and place it in your mouth for a specified time. You can sleep with the 10% solution, which must be used for at least 6 hours a day, but the 22% solution is so strong that it can only be worn 1 hour a day. The process takes 2 to 3 weeks, and your dentist will monitor you weekly to be sure you're getting the best results without harming your gums. Bleaching isn't permanent—your teeth will darken over time—but the trays can be reused, under your dentist's supervision, for touch-ups.

The in-office procedure is quicker, but less effective. Your dentist shields your gums and lips, then applies a highly concentrated gel (a 30% to 35% solution of hydrogen peroxide) to your teeth. Next, he uses either a laser or a power light to activate the gel. It takes 1 to 2 hours to treat your entire mouth, but you may need 3 visits to get the best outcome. For optimum results in the shortest time, your dentist can combine in-office bleaching with 3 to 4 days of at-home treatment to lock in the color.

ask the experts

What should I consider when deciding on bleaching?

Not all tooth stains are easily treatable. Discolorations that are the result of high fever or the use of certain medications are difficult to bleach out completely. With laser or power bleaching, you abstain from intensely colored foods (red wine, coffee, grape juice) for 24 hours following treatment. If you use the at-home method, you'll have to stay away from those foods as well as cigarettes throughout the entire 2- or 3-week process.

Are there any drawbacks to bleaching?

The gel may cause painful gum irritation and teeth may temporarily be sensitive to heat and cold. Bleaching will leave a noticeable color difference wherever there are cracks in the teeth and, if you have receding gums and your roots are exposed, at the gum line. Also, teeth that have been capped or bonded will not respond to bleaching.

How long will the results last?

Unfortunately, there is no way to bleach your teeth permanently. The color will usually begin to fade slightly in the first 2 weeks after treatment, then stabilize for 6 months to 2 years, depending in part on the foods you eat (drinking red wine will soon undo the brighter white). No matter which method you use, the process will have to be repeated in 1 to 2 years.

What about over-the-counter bleaching products?

Over-the-counter products, which sell for around $50, work the same as at-home systems—minus your dentist's supervision. The one-size-fits-all tray available in these kits isn't as effective as a custom-fitted one from your dentist. And, the less perfect the fit, the more chance your gums have of becoming irritated or even burned from uneven contact with the bleaching gel.

FEES

Bleaching

In-office laser or power bleaching using the strongest solution (35% hydrogen peroxide) costs from $500 to $1,500. At-home bleaching, which uses a less intense solution of carbamide peroxide, runs from $300 to $800. The price includes the gel, tray, and dentist's fee for weekly monitoring of the process.

contour a new look

Shape up your smile

With aesthetic contouring, your dentist can provide maximum improvement in the appearance of your teeth with minimal pain—to your mouth or your wallet. Here, your dentist is zeroing in on the shape of your teeth. Reshaping teeth to make them look smoother, more uniform, and more evenly spaced can make a dramatic difference. And since the treatment, which is done with a drill, sandpaper discs, and polishing wheels, removes such a small amount of tooth structure, an anesthetic is usually not needed.

Contouring can be used to shorten teeth, remove chips on the bottom edges of teeth to make them look even again, and round out pointy teeth. It can also reduce the width of teeth, which can correct a common smile imperfection—having two overly wide front teeth that overlap the adjacent teeth. Aesthetic contouring is most commonly used to even out some lower teeth that may appear higher than others due to crowding.

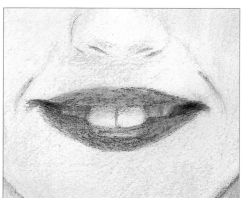 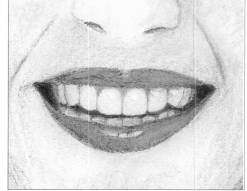

Your dentist can reshape your teeth to create a more uniform—and attractive—appearance.

ask the experts

Are there any risks associated with this process?

You may experience sensitivity to heat and cold, but the sensitivity should subside over time.

How long will the results last?

Your new contouring should last a lifetime.

I'm a 24-year-old woman and I have been told that my teeth look like a man's! Can anything be done?

There are, in fact, gender differences in teeth. Women's teeth tend to be rounded at the corners, while men's are usually more squared off. Aesthetic contouring can be used to reshape your teeth to make them appear more feminine or masculine.

FEES

Aesthetic Contouring

This is the least expensive of all cosmetic dental procedures. Depending on how extensive the work you're having done is, contouring can cost anywhere from $100 to $1,000 for the whole mouth.

bonding

Makeovers for odd teeth, changing surface color, and more

The bonding process is a fix for teeth—mainly front teeth—that have serious stains and other imperfections. Basically, it involves a putty-like material that is chemically adhered to a tooth. Here's how it works: Your dentist etches a tooth (similar to etching glass) with phosphoric acid to remove the shine or glaze of the enamel so that other material will adhere to that tooth. Then he applies a **composite resin** (a medical-grade plastic) that seeps into the now open areas of enamel, and exposes that resin to a high-intensity light. The light causes a chemical reaction within the resin, which then hardens, seals off the enamel that has been opened up, and bonds to the tooth surface. The dentist then uses instruments to polish and contour the resin into the desired shape.

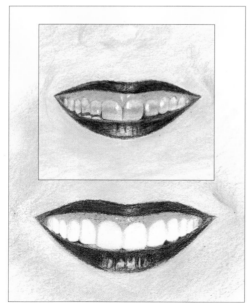

In addition to changing the shade of your teeth, bonding can repair a chip or fracture, or build up or otherwise alter the shape of a tooth (for example, you can lengthen a short tooth). This same composite material can be used in fillings for those who prefer to match their tooth color. It can also help camouflage stains—see left for before and after illustration.

In general, bonding doesn't require an anesthetic, and the results are immediate—and reversible. If, for example, your teeth were bonded to change their color and you're unhappy with the result, you can remove the bonding material and your tooth structure will be relatively intact.

ask the experts

How long does bonding last?

Bonding will generally last from 3 to 10 years before you need to repair or redo the work. The resin can chip, and it picks up stains and plaque, which sticks easily to bonding material. Also, because bonding material is opaque—unlike enamel, which is clear and shining—it dulls over time. Because it requires a great deal of maintenance and repair it may not be the best long-term economic option for cosmetic purposes.

FEES

Bonding

Along with aesthetic contouring, bonding is a cost-effective way to improve your smile. Prices vary depending on the extent of the work you're having done. They generally range from $100 to $600 per tooth.

CAUTIONARY TALE

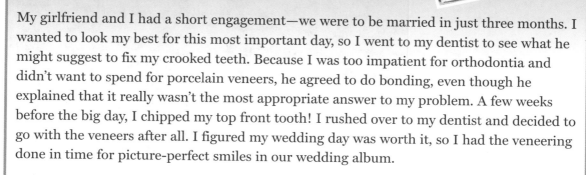

A chip off the old block(head)

My girlfriend and I had a short engagement—we were to be married in just three months. I wanted to look my best for this most important day, so I went to my dentist to see what he might suggest to fix my crooked teeth. Because I was too impatient for orthodontia and didn't want to spend for porcelain veneers, he agreed to do bonding, even though he explained that it really wasn't the most appropriate answer to my problem. A few weeks before the big day, I chipped my top front tooth! I rushed over to my dentist and decided to go with the veneers after all. I figured my wedding day was worth it, so I had the veneering done in time for picture-perfect smiles in our wedding album.

Stu E., Flint, Michigan

veneers

How to get a movie star smile

Veneers are the pinnacle of cosmetic dentistry, and can correct a myriad of tooth problems. Veneers are custom-made, thin porcelain or composite **laminates** (resin shells) that are bonded to tooth enamel—imagine very thin fake fingernails glued onto your front teeth.

Veneers are not only more effective than bleaching for whitening teeth, they can also change the shape of teeth better than contouring or bonding (and are much stronger than bonding). **Porcelain veneers** (those made of a ceramic, tooth-colored material) reflect light like natural enamel so they look more lifelike and retain their luster better than bonding material. Veneers can close up spaces between teeth and even make crooked teeth appear to be perfectly straight, camouflaging flaws that weren't permanently corrected with braces.

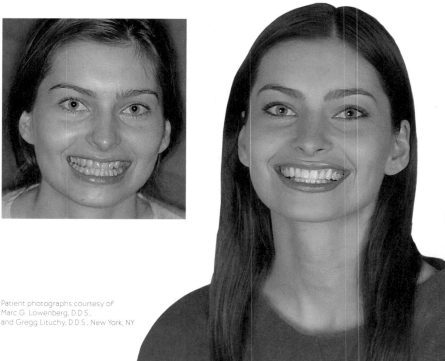

Patient photographs courtesy of
Marc G. Lowenberg, D.D.S.,
and Gregg Lituchy, D.D.S., New York, NY

Your dentist removes a half-millimeter of enamel from the front surface of the tooth (the veneer itself is more than a millimeter thick). Then, he etches the tooth with phosphoric acid, as in the bonding process (see page 104), and applies a resin cement to the tooth and the veneer, which bonds the veneer to the enamel. The process takes at least 2 visits to complete. Unlike bonding, veneering with porcelain is irreversible, so you'll have to touch up or redo your veneers over time, usually every 5 to 10 years.

ask the experts

Can veneers give me a sexier or more youthful smile?

Your dentist can give you a sexy smile by using veneers to make a narrow smile look wider by filling in spaces and building out your teeth. *Voila*! You're flashing a wide, Julia Roberts or Whitney Houston grin. Veneers can also reverse your aging smile by lengthening worn-down upper teeth and making them thicker so they give more support to thinning lips.

What risks are associated with this procedure?

Since veneers permanently alter tooth structure, remember that you're committing to a lifetime of maintenance. And, as with any dental work in which part of a tooth is removed, you run the risk of inflaming the nerve.

FEES

Veneers

Veneers range in price from $400 to $2,000 per tooth, depending on how extensive the work is and whether the material used is porcelain or composite.

braces for grown-ups

A tried-and-true method gets a new approach

Years ago, an orthodontist focused solely on making teeth fit together perfectly. Today, when deciding on a treatment, orthodontists take into consideration not only the structure of your teeth, but also the curves and angles of your face and jawline to achieve better harmony. This could mean recommending braces or even jaw restructuring (for more on this see page 110).

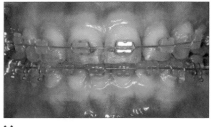

You don't have to look like you have a mouth full of metal. Clear braces are much less noticeable.

Your orthodontist takes X-rays and impressions to create plaster models of your teeth, then constructs braces by cementing or bonding brackets to the teeth and affixing wires to the brackets. These wires will need adjusting about every 6 weeks throughout the course of treatment. Traditional metal braces are the most durable and the least expensive. **Ceramic** (clear) braces are more brittle than metal and are pricier, too.

Lingual braces, next in cost, are metal braces fitted along the inside of the teeth so that they're hidden. (They cost more in part because they are more difficult and time intensive to install.) Because they're closer to the tongue they're more difficult to adapt to—a fact you'll be acutely aware of the first few times you try to speak or eat with them.

Invisalign is a state-of-the-art product that consists of removable, snap-on plastic trays, or tooth aligners, that are custom-fitted to your teeth. The aligners, which exert a controlled force on the teeth, are changed every two weeks to move the teeth into a new position. This technology is best for people who want to straighten crooked or crowded teeth, but who have an overall good bite that will not require much jaw movement to correct. The cost falls somewhere between ceramic and lingual braces.

Removable appliances (retainers, springs), which are for mild cases and usually worn only at night, are the least expensive.

ask the experts

How long does treatment take?

Treatment varies depending on what's being corrected, but in general lasts 2 to 2½ years. Removable appliances typically take more time.

Are there any risks associated with this process?

TMJ (temporomandibular, or jaw joint) problems, which can include pain or clicking sounds, may be triggered or worsened. Orthodontists debate whether the use of orthodontics causes—or cures—TMJ.

What other considerations are there?

You'll feel physically uncomfortable and socially awkward at first. Also, you'll need to make time for orthodontist appointments over the course of treatment and follow up after the braces come off.

How old is too old or how young too young for braces?

From age 7 on, anyone can get braces. (Today's conventional wisdom is, the earlier the intervention, the better.) And you're never too old to have braces if your teeth, gums, and bone are healthy.

How long will the results last?

Teeth will shift over time unless you keep wearing your retainer, a removable device given to you when the braces come off, to be worn at night. The retainer keeps your teeth in their new position. Want a guarantee that your teeth won't shift over time? Consider a bonded retainer—a small wire that is affixed behind your top or bottom front teeth—which can be left in place for years.

FEES

Braces

Costs run between $4,000 and $8,000 for the duration of treatment, depending on the kind of braces you are getting and the severity of the condition you are treating. Lingual (inner surface) braces can cost even more, up to $9,000; removable appliances, which may be all you require, can be as inexpensive as $500. Some orthodontia is covered by insurance, so check your dental plan.

jaw restructuring

Consider your profile before undertaking other facial cosmetic surgery

Oral surgery is all about proportion. The face can be divided into thirds (from the forehead into the eyebrows, the brows to below the nose, and below the nose to the chin), and those thirds should be proportional. Oral surgeons, working with general dentists and orthodontists, can help you achieve this facial harmony. An oral surgeon can address what is out of proportion by repositioning your chin and jaw. For example, you may be considering a nose job because you think your nose sticks out too far when the real imbalance could be corrected by having surgery to bring your recessed jaw forward.

The first step to jaw surgery usually begins with a visit to your dentist or orthodontist. Maybe you're unhappy with the way your mouth looks, but you may not realize the appearance is off because your jaw is in the wrong position and that it can be best corrected by surgery. Or perhaps you want to change your profile, which means altering the skeletal shape of your face.

Once the jaw is in the desired position, your surgeon will wire it shut for 6 weeks or stabilize it with screws to permit you to open and close your mouth.

Jaw reconstruction is usually performed in a hospital, under general anesthesia. The jaw is repositioned by cutting and sliding the upper or lower jawbone and placing it in proper **occlusion** (a bite in which the top and bottom teeth meet perfectly). Your oral surgeon can also expand the jaw, or move the chin backward, forward or sideways.

ask the experts

What risks exist with this procedure?

Paresthesia, which is a numbness or loss of sensation, can occur if the surgeon accidentally cuts a nerve. This is more likely to happen with work on the lower jaw, where you can lose some of the feeling beneath the lip or on the chin. Fear not: Since motor function wouldn't be affected, you won't wind up with a drooling problem or a paralyzed lip. Also, **TMJ** (temporomandibular, or jaw joint) problems could be triggered by jaw surgery.

What is recovery like?

Your jaw may remain wired shut for 6 weeks, limiting you to a liquid diet. If your jaw is fixed with screws, you'll be able to open your mouth, but you'll be restricted to a soft diet. Expect lots of swelling, with the worst of it over in a few weeks; minor swelling can last for 6 months or more. You can return to work in 10 days, but it will be 4 to 6 weeks before you can resume strenuous activities. You'll have follow-up visits with your oral surgeon to remove the wiring and check your bite, and with your orthodontist or general dentist to address any other tooth-alignment or cosmetic matters.

What other considerations are there?

Your appearance may change dramatically, so you must be prepared psychologically for the new you (see page 12). Taking certain anti-clotting medications or having diabetes could be obstacles to your having the procedure.

What age is too young for jaw restructuring?

The surgery isn't recommended for anyone who is still growing. The minimum age is 16 for girls and 18 for boys.

FEES

Jaw Restructuring

Insurance coverage for jaw surgery depends on the severity of the **malocclusion** (bad bite). The worse the bite, the greater the chance that insurance will pay for the "usual and customary" portion of the surgery. The cost is about $7,000 to $8,000 for a single jaw, and upward of $10,000 if both the upper and lower jaws are worked on.

now what do I do?

My smile is all gums. Is there a fix for my gummy grin?

A general dentist can use a laser or more conventional instruments to remove some gum tissue, thereby exposing more of the teeth as well as evening out the gum line. The cost of a **laser gingivectomy** (gum tissue removal, also known as a **gum lift**) ranges from $1,000 to $2,000 for the whole mouth.

What can I do about my embarrassing receding gums?

If you've lost a lot of gum tissue, which can make your lower front teeth appear longer than they should be at the root surface, a periodontist can graft new tissue over the area to cover the exposed surface. The procedure can cost anywhere from $450 to $950 per tooth.

I need fillings in my front teeth, but I don't want a tin grin. What are my options?

Today, silver fillings are being replaced with tooth-colored porcelain and composite materials, which are bonded to the tooth. Porcelain most closely mimics natural tooth enamel, and because it's an inert substance, there's no concern over toxicity as some believe is the case with the mercury in silver fillings. Porcelain comes in numerous shades; your dentist will pick the one that most closely matches your tooth color. Porcelain fillings can cost from $400 to $1,500 per tooth. Since nothing lasts forever, expect to have to redo these restorations in 10 to 15 years.

What's the best way to replace a tooth that's been knocked out?

For a front tooth, you should consider having a single tooth implant along with veneering on the adjacent teeth to improve the overall aesthetic. The implant is done in two steps: First your dentist will implant, or bury, a titanium root form in the bone under your gum. This must then "take" to the bone over the next 4 to 6 months. During this time you'll wear a temporary tooth-like cap. Then your dentist will screw a post into the implant and place a final cap, or crown, over the post. The cost of an implant ranges from $2,000 to $4,500, depending on the extent of the work you're having done and whether you're also getting veneers.

What if I can't have an implant to replace my missing tooth?

Not everyone is a candidate for, or chooses to have, implants. In this case, your dentist can use a **bridge**, which literally bridges the space of a missing tooth by putting caps on either side of the space, and another in the empty pocket. He or she then cements all three together. The price of a bridge varies with how many teeth are being replaced, but is generally between $3,000 and $6,000.

If I have bridges, can I still get orthodontia to straighten my teeth?

Because bridges adhere two or more teeth together, they can resist tooth movement. An orthodontist will be able to determine if your bridges would interfere with successful treatment or whether orthodontia would damage your bridgework.

Now where do I go?!

CONTACTS

American Academy of
Cosmetic Dentistry
www.aacd.com
800-543-9220

Academy of General Dentistry
www.agd.org
312-440-4300

American Association of
Orthodontists
www.braces.org
800-STRAIGHT

American Academy
of Facial Plastic
and Reconstructive Surgery
www.aafprs.org
800-332-FACE

ADDITIONAL INFORMATION

Braces: A Consumer's Guide to Orthodontics
By G. Ray Callahan, D.D.S.

Chapter 7

Breasts and Chests

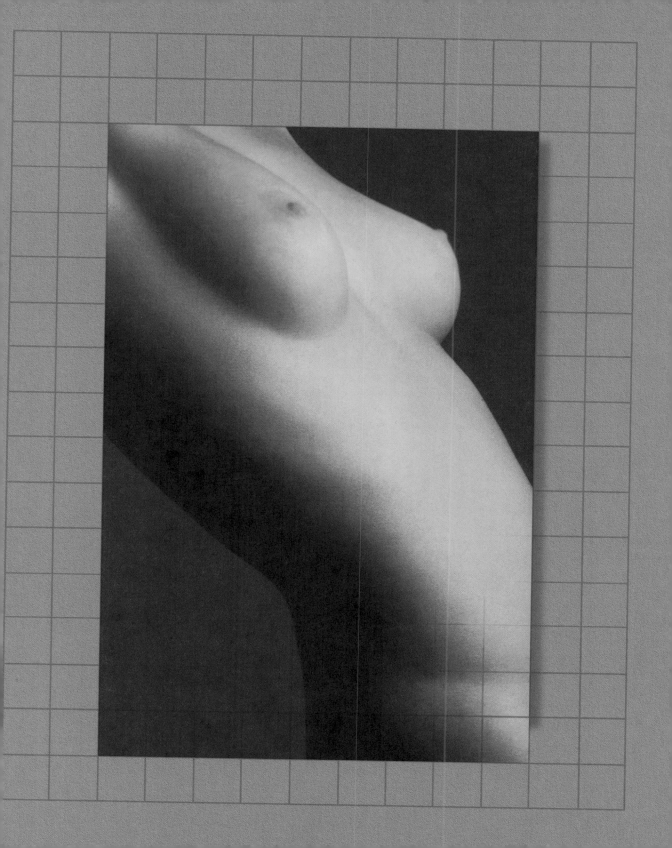

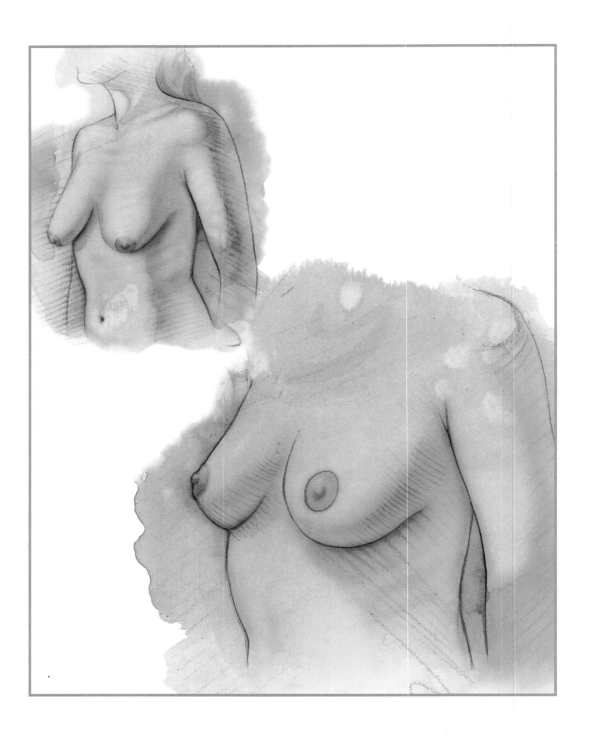

What takes most people by surprise is how the size and shape of breasts can change over time. Weight loss and gain, pregnancy, and age all have a huge impact on how breasts look. Cosmetic surgery can restore, enhance, or reduce what you have now—for men, too.

need a lift?

What a breast lift can do for you

Thanks to age, pregnancy, and weight loss, breasts sag. One solution is a **breast lift**, or **mastopexy**, which involves moving the nipple and **areola** (the pigmented skin around the nipple) back to a higher, more youthful position and, at the same time, reshaping the breast. This will raise sagging breasts—for a time. There is no technique that will defy gravity indefinitely, just as there is no stopping the aging process, though you can control weight fluctuations, which also take a toll on breast lifts over time.

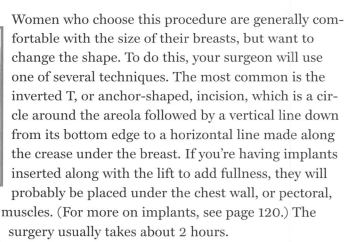

Women who choose this procedure are generally comfortable with the size of their breasts, but want to change the shape. To do this, your surgeon will use one of several techniques. The most common is the inverted T, or anchor-shaped, incision, which is a circle around the areola followed by a vertical line down from its bottom edge to a horizontal line made along the crease under the breast. If you're having implants inserted along with the lift to add fullness, they will probably be placed under the chest wall, or pectoral, muscles. (For more on implants, see page 120.) The surgery usually takes about 2 hours.

The success of this procedure depends on several factors: the elasticity of your skin, your age, overall health, and the size and shape of your breasts and body. Also, each doctor will give you a look that is in keeping with his aesthetic. Ask your doctor to show you books with examples of the work he has done so that you can see breasts and bodies similar to your own in "before" and "after" photos.

ask the experts

What happens after the surgery? What is recovery like?

You will feel sore, swollen, and bruised in the breast area for the first two days. You can expect some loss of feeling in your nipples and breast skin, caused by the swelling after surgery, but this should fade, along with the incision scars, over the next few weeks. While you can return to work within a week, you will not be able to do heavy lifting or upper-body exercises for another 3 weeks. Then you can slowly start back into your regular routine. But listen to your body—it will let you know when you are overdoing it.

What are the risks associated with this type of procedure?

A breast lift can occasionally result in loss of sensation in your nipples or breasts, as well as **asymmetry**, or uneven breasts. You will have permanent scars, but they are usually positioned to be hidden by clothing and should fade over time. Note to smokers: You may not heal as well, and often have wider scars (as if you needed another reason to quit!).

How long will the results last?

Unless you frequently gain and lose lots of weight, or you become pregnant, you should not need a second procedure for 10 to 15 years or longer.

Can I nurse if I have a breast lift?

Yes. A mastopexy typically will not interfere with breast-feeding, since your milk ducts and nipples are left intact.

FEES

Breast Lift

Surgeons' fees alone range from $3,000 to $8,000. A lift is not covered by insurance unless it is for a particular medical circumstance, such as breast reconstruction after breast cancer treatment, a birth defect, or an injury (see breast reconstruction on page 126).

implants

What they are and how they work

There are two kinds of implants: **silicone** and **saline**. Silicone is a polymer that can be produced in a variety of forms, including the rubbery shell and the gel filling that is used for a breast implant. A saline implant has a silicone shell that is filled with sterile salt water.

There are four types of saline implants to choose from: smooth, textured, teardrop (also known as anatomically shaped), and round. And there are combinations of the four. The most commonly used are the round, smooth implants.

The two major manufacturers of implants offer warranty coverage in case of rupture (see next page). Implants usually last 10 to 20 years, after which time they might shift or are likely to leak. Expect to replace them at least once, and perhaps supplement them with a breast lift (see page 118) as gravity and aging take their toll.

Both saline and silicone implants can rupture and leak. While there have been no health risks associated with ruptured saline implants, ruptured silicone implants have been under scrutiny since concerns were raised in the early '90s about their possible connection to autoimmune conditions. To date, there has been no evidence to prove these allegations. However, while continuing to study this matter, the FDA has ruled that only breast reconstruction and implant revision patients can receive silicone implants.

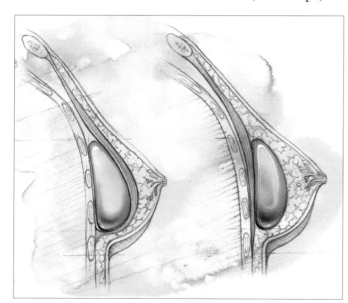

Implants can be positioned behind the chest muscle or in front of it.

ask the experts

Are there warranties on implants?

Yes, there are, and you can get them directly from the two major makers of implants. If the implants rupture at any time, they will replace them for free. If they break within the first 5 years, they will reimburse a portion of the operating costs to replace them. You can even get an extended warranty.

What can I do if I'm not satisfied with my implants?

If you're not happy with the implants, remedying that will depend on what you're unhappy with. Is it the size? The position? The shape? The most common lament among women is that their breasts aren't large enough, which can be resolved by inserting larger implants.

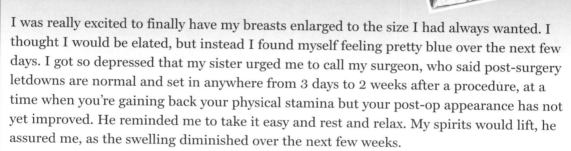

CAUTIONARY TALE

There is no instant beauty

I was really excited to finally have my breasts enlarged to the size I had always wanted. I thought I would be elated, but instead I found myself feeling pretty blue over the next few days. I got so depressed that my sister urged me to call my surgeon, who said post-surgery letdowns are normal and set in anywhere from 3 days to 2 weeks after a procedure, at a time when you're gaining back your physical stamina but your post-op appearance has not yet improved. He reminded me to take it easy and rest and relax. My spirits would lift, he assured me, as the swelling diminished over the next few weeks.

Elizabeth S., Evanston, Illinois

bigger breasts

Opting for implants

Breast **augmentation**, or enlargement, is for women who want to increase their bustline by one or more cup sizes. This procedure can help if you wish to increase your normal breast size or to restore fullness lost after pregnancy, to balance a difference in breast size, or as a reconstructive technique after breast surgery. (Read more about breast reconstruction on page 126.)

The surgery calls for the insertion of **saline** (salt water)-filled implants into the breasts. Most surgeons position implants behind the chest wall, or pectoral, muscles (**submuscular**). This results in more accurate mammograms and may reduce infection and **capsular contracture** (hardening of the tissue around the implants), so the implants will stay softer. The procedure lasts from one to several hours.

An implant comes flat. The surgeon rolls it up like a cigar and typically inserts it through a small incision made in your armpit, the lower edge of the **areola** (the pigmented skin around the nipple), or in the crease of the lower part of your breast. He then uses a tube to fill it with sterile saline, expanding it to the size you want.

Keep in mind that while an implant will do a great deal to fill up your breast, if you have very loose or sagging skin you may also need a breast lift for a good result (see page 118 for more on breast lifts). Otherwise, your nipple may end up sitting too low.

Note: Silicone implants are available primarily to women who need breast reconstruction or implant revision. (See page 120 for more info on silicone versus saline implants.)

FEES

Implants

Surgeons' fees alone range from $3,000 to $6,000. Unless the implants are necessary for breast reconstruction due to cancer or another trauma, this is considered a purely cosmetic procedure and is not covered by insurance.

ask the experts

What are the risks associated with this type of procedure?

Among the risks specific to implant surgery are **asymmetry** (uneven breasts or nipples), **deflation** (saline implants can rupture and deflate), **hematoma** (a collection of blood around the implant), poor scarring, changes in nipple sensation (it may decrease, disappear altogether, or even become too intense), and **capsular contracture** (a tightening of the scar tissue the body forms around the implant). Also, if the surgeon has to cut the milk ducts, breast-feeding may no longer be possible.

What is recovery like?

For the first 48 hours you'll be given pain medication and wrapped in a light dressing. Though you'll feel sore and bruised for 2 weeks, your breasts will be swollen for months. Post-op care varies from doctor to doctor, with some having you wear a surgical bra (no underwire!) or compression bandage for days, others for weeks, and still others none at all. Figure on 2 to 3 months before you can resume regular activity.

If I want larger breasts, should I get a lift or implants?

If anything, a lift will make your breasts appear slightly smaller. A lift can improve the shape of the breast by tightening the skin and moving the nipple higher. But if you want to make the breasts bigger, you will need to have implants.

Do I still need to get mammograms on a regular basis?

Yes! And you must tell the technician about your implants to be sure she takes extra views (a typical screening mammogram includes only two views). Implants do render mammograms less accurate in detecting cancer, but they may detect implant ruptures or leakage. Some doctors may suggest you have an **MRI** (magnetic resonance imaging) for a better read.

breast reduction

When bigger isn't better

Breast reduction may be necessary if you suffer from **macro-mastia** (very large, heavy breasts). This condition can create serious neck and back pain and rashes under the breast. Bras at this size are cumbersome contraptions. You may also be caught in a Catch-22: While you would benefit from exercise to lose weight, which would likely reduce the weight in the breasts, your breasts can be too big to exercise comfortably.

Psychological issues also come into play. Many women with heavy, sagging breasts feel they can't participate in various activities or wear stylish clothing because it makes them feel self-conscious.

To reduce breast size, your surgeon may simply use **lipo-suction** to minimize scarring (see page 138 for more about liposuction, the use of which in the breasts is controversial). If you are not a candidate for that, he can perform a breast reduction. The most common technique involves an upside-down T, or anchor, incision, which follows the natural contour of the breast. With extremely large breasts, the nipple and **areola** (the pigmented skin around the nipple) will likely have to be taken off and reattached, like a graft, once the breasts have been reduced.

The procedure can result in some degree of scarring around the nipple, and down and under the breast.

ask the experts

What risks are associated with this type of procedure?

The disappointing results can be **asymmetry** (uneven breasts) or poor scarring, which can mean anything from a thickening of the scar to very bad **keloids**, aka "scar tumors" because of the way they grow outside the incision site. The worst complication is the loss of the nipple and/or areola, which may occur if blood flow cannot be established in the newly reattached tissue. There is also no guarantee that sensation or the ability to nurse will be restored.

Realistically, what can I expect from this surgery?

Despite the extensive scarring that results from this procedure, women who opt for breast reduction are often the happiest among those who have had any type of breast surgery. This is because the scarring often pales before the pain and discomfort they endured before having their weighty breasts reduced.

What happens after the surgery? What is recovery like?

You'll be wrapped in gauze dressings and a compression garment for 1 to 2 days, then moved to a surgical or sports bra (no underwire!). Pain should be minimal. You'll wear the surgical bra for up to 3 weeks, round the clock. You can expect some loss of feeling in your nipples and breast skin, caused by the swelling after surgery, but this should fade as the swelling subsides over the next few weeks. In some women, however, it can last a year or more, or even be permanent.

FEES

Breast Reduction

Breast reduction is frequently covered by insurance. While pre-approval is required, this procedure is usually recognized as being medically necessary due to the pain, discomfort, and related conditions that very heavy breasts can cause. Generally, the surgeon's fee for breast reduction ranges from $5,000 to $10,000.

breast reconstruction

Ready for the new you

Women and men who have a deformity in the breast area (from cancer treatment, trauma, or birth defects) are candidates for breast reconstruction. This procedure can be done for one or both breasts and at any age. Breast reconstruction involves, literally, reconstructing what's been taken away. In most cases that is the breast mound itself and the **nipple/areolar complex** (the nipple and the pigmented ring of skin around it).

There are two basic techniques in reconstruction: using your own tissue or inserting an implant. If you use your own tissue (typically fatty tissue, muscle, and skin from the stomach, back, buttocks, or thighs), you'll have the closest match to your breast tissue. But this option means having two surgery sites and two scars—one from the **mastectomy** (removal of the breast) and and the other from where the additional tissue was taken.

Having a breast implant (see page 122) is a less involved operation. However, there needs to be enough tissue to cover it. Following a mastectomy, this is often not the case, so a technique called **tissue expansion** is used to stretch the skin to create more coverage in the breast area first. Here, an **expander** implant is inserted flat and then over several office visits is slowly inflated with **saline** (sterile salt water) until the appropriate size is reached. The expander implant is then removed and replaced with a regular breast implant. Breast reconstruction patients have a choice about the type of implant they can have: saline or silicone (see page 120 for more on implants).

Nipple/areola reconstruction, usually done as a follow-up procedure using local anesthesia, completes the breast reconstruction. The coloration is matched with tattooing (see page 64 for more on tattooing).

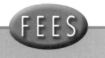

FEES

Breast Reconstruction

Surgeons' fees alone range from $3,500 to $10,000, depending on how much work needs to be done—one or both breasts, for example. Reconstruction should be fully covered, but insurers still deny some procedures, so be prepared to do battle for complete coverage, especially if you will require a surgical adjustment to a remaining healthy breast so that your breasts match.

ask the experts

Should I get an implant right after my mastectomy?

This is a question that you must discuss thoroughly with the doctor who is handling your cancer treatment. There is some debate about whether immediate or delayed reconstruction is better psychologically and emotionally. Immediate reconstruction may spare a woman from having to cope with having no breast at all. But some doctors advise waiting to allow patients time to grieve over the loss of a body part and have real closure, then move on to reconstruction in a better frame of mind.

If I have only one breast removed and reconstructed, will it look like my other breast?

Breasts are paired, so your surgeon will need to make the two match as best he can. If the remaining healthy breast is very large, for example, or sagging from age, this may mean undergoing a breast reduction (see page 124) or a breast lift (see page 118) on that breast in order to create symmetry between it and the reconstructed breast. Also, differences between your breasts can appear over time. For example, your natural breast will continue to age and sag, but a breast reconstructed with an implant will not change, so symmetry will not be maintained. This may require cosmetic adjustments (a breast lift, for example) to the healthy breast over the years.

What happens if cancer recurs after having had breast reconstruction?

Your reconstructed breast should not interfere with further cancer treatment, but you will have to have the procedure repeated because radiation will adversely affect the reconstructed breast. The good news: If you have not had a local recurrence within a year, it is not likely to happen at all.

Online Shopping

These online stores have a number of garments and bras for post-operative and mastectomy situations:

www.bralady.com

www.brafitters.com

www.bodygraphicbras.com

www.judysintimate apparel.com

www.buststop.com

www.victoriassecret.com

pec implants for men

A chest Tarzan would envy

Pectoralis implants, or implants in the muscle area of the chest wall, are gaining in popularity among bodybuilders and non-bodybuilders alike, particularly on the West Coast. How does this procedure work?

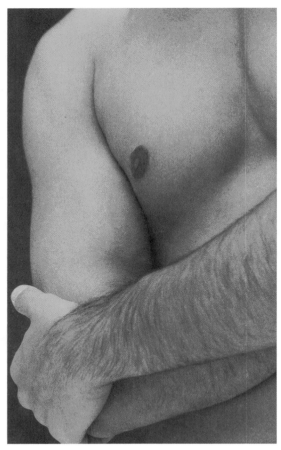

Your surgeon will either use a preformed silicone block—they come in several shapes—or he can carve the implant if that will fit you best. Breast implants for men are made of solid silicone, so there is nothing to leak, unlike a silicone gel-filled implant for a woman. (For more on silicone and safety, see page 120.) Then your surgeon will likely make an incision in the armpit, to avoid having a scar on the breast. The implant is placed in a pocket underneath the pectoral muscle, on top of the rib cage.

Good skin elasticity is important, but less so than for a woman having breast **augmentation**, or enlargement, due to the nature of the implant, its shape, and where it will sit. However, you do need to be in decent shape for this to be effective. If you have loose skin on your chest as a result of having been very overweight, this implant will not fill it up.

@sk the experts

What risks are associated with this type of procedure?

Asymmetry (uneven pecs) is a significant risk. Another is the hardening of the tissue around the implant, called **capsular contracture**. This is less likely to occur with men than women who have had a breast enlargement because the implants for men are firmer. Poor scarring can also result. The worst complication, however, would be tissue loss. Because the blood supply has been weakened by the surgery, the nipple and/or **areola** (pigmented skin around the nipple) may be lost, and require reconstruction.

What happens after the surgery? What is recovery like?

You will feel sore, swollen, and bruised for a few days. For the first couple of days, you will have a light dressing, then tape on your chest for about 5 days. Unlike a woman who has had a breast enlargement, you won't have to wear a compression garment because the pocket for the implant is smaller and there is little to shift around. You will be able to return to work in 3 to 5 days. You will have to avoid heavy lifting and vigorous exercise for about a month, to prevent the risk of bleeding.

FEES

Pec Implants

Surgeons' fees alone range from $3,000 to $6,000. A chest wall deformity that requires this procedure will be covered by insurance.

breast reduction for men

The one place you don't want to be big

FEES

Male Breast Reduction

Male breast reduction is generally not covered by insurance unless it is performed in adolescence (17 to 18 years old). Most insurance companies reason that if you have lived with the condition for many years, you are not psychologically challenged by it as a mature man. There are three types of procedures, which vary in complexity. For a mild case requiring only liposuction, the surgeon's fees alone range from $2,500 to $5,000. To treat a case of moderate breast enlargement, requiring liposuction and cutting out tissue, the costs range from $4,500 to $6,500. For severe enlargement, the surgeon's fees range from $5,000 to $8,000.

Many men suffer from **gynecomastia**, or enlarged male breasts. The term is derived from the Greek words for "woman-like breasts." This condition occurs in 40% to 60% of the male population. It can affect just one breast, or both. It generally starts in puberty, when hormone changes can trigger growth of breast tissue and fat.

Your surgeon will decide which of the three common techniques to use during the hour-and-a-half operation based on the degree of your breast enlargement. For mild cases, he will simply use **liposuction** to remove the fat (see page 138 for more on liposuction). For men who have moderate breast enlargement, your surgeon may combine liposuction to remove the fat with surgery to remove breast tissue. In severe cases, particularly if you are very overweight, your surgeon may opt for a direct excision, or cutting out, of breast tissue, fat; and skin from the center, sides, and bottom of each breast (resulting in very visible scarring).

Before a surgeon will perform a male breast reduction procedure, he will ask you for a thorough medical history and give you a physical to rule out possible causes of the enlarged breasts. This can include a tumor, such as a testicular or adrenal tumor, which may be producing hormones that spur breast growth, as well as various drugs, such as marijuana, excess alcohol, steroids, and diuretics (for example, Lasix), which, if stopped, may make the breast enlargement disappear. If you are very overweight and have not first tried to correct the problem through diet and exercise, your doctor may not proceed with the surgery until you do. The best candidates are those who have firm, elastic skin that will reshape to the body's new contours.

ask the experts

What risks are associated with this type of procedure?

In addition to the general risks associated with any surgery—infection, skin injury, excessive bleeding, adverse reaction to anesthesia—the disappointing results with male breast reduction can include **asymmetry** (uneven breasts), noticeable scarring (especially with surgery for severe enlargement), sensation changes and numbness, permanent pigment changes in the breast area, **seroma** (fluid collection under the skin, which is common with liposuction) or **hematoma** (a collection of blood under the skin). Also, if too much tissue and fat are removed, you'll end up with a collapsed or concave look to the chest.

Realistically, what can I expect from this surgery? How long will the results last?

Male breast reduction can certainly improve your self-image, not to mention your appearance. This procedure is usually required just once in a lifetime. However, if you gain a great deal of weight, you can bring on a recurrence.

What happens after the surgery? What is recovery like?

You will have to wear a compression garment continuously for 2 to 3 weeks to keep the skin in place and to avoid fluid or blood collection under the skin. You may be required to wear this garment for several more weeks at night. Expect to be quite sore for a couple of weeks, and swollen and bruised for as long as several months. At first, your breasts will appear to be as large as ever, due to the swelling, and they will feel hard. It will take about 6 to 8 weeks before your breasts soften and feel more natural. After 3 months the swelling will be appreciably less. You'll be able to resume light activity—walking around—after a day or two, and will be able to return to work within a few days. You will have to avoid heavy exercise or sports for 3 or 4 weeks.

now what do I do?

Answers to common questions

How do I know what size to become?

Bring a picture from a magazine or bathing suit catalog to your surgeon when you first meet. Talking cup size leaves you both open to interpretation since bra sizes vary from brand to brand, but a visual image shows your doctor exactly what you envision will be attractive for you. Also, go over pre- and post-op pictures in your doctor's office. Be sure to look for women with a body similar to your own, to get a better idea of what the procedure would look like for you. Be cautious about what you might see on an imaging system, or computer simulation, if your surgeon offers it. Computers can mislead by creating beautiful breasts that may not work for your body shape, nor can they predict how you will heal.

What must I do regarding sun exposure after a cosmetic surgery procedure?

From the day of surgery for 6 months or longer, depending on the procedure you have, you will have to avoid exposure to the sun. Sunlight can permanently affect the skin's pigmentation, causing the scars from surgery to turn dark. Worse, strong sunlight can burn the surgery area's scars and sensitive skin without your realizing it, causing an injury as severe as a third-degree burn. If sun exposure is unavoidable, use a strong sunblock, wear light-colored clothing (black absorbs heat), and stay as covered up as possible.

Can implants interfere with the detection of breast cancer?

You must tell your mammographer that you have had implants so that she can take additional screening views of your breasts. Saline implants allow X-ray beams to pass right through them, so they don't interfere with mammograms as much as the denser silicone. Your doctor may have you get an **MRI** (magnetic resonance imaging), if he or she feels a better read is called for.

Could implants leave me with rippling or wrinkling?

This is one of the more common problems with implants. There are certain areas where the breast tissue is thinner and you can see the indents or feel rippling under the skin. It occurs more often in thinner, smaller breasts. Unfortunately, nothing can be done for this.

I heard implants can make noise. Is that true?

Saline implants have been known to make sloshing, gurgling, popping, crackling, or even humming sounds. These should diminish as your breast tissue molds around the implants. While the sounds may be awkward, don't panic—it does not mean your implants are leaking.

Now where do I go?!

CONTACTS

American Society
of Plastic Surgeons
www.plasticsurgery.org
847-228-9900

American Society for
Aesthetic Plastic Surgery
www.surgery.org
212-921-0500

ADDITIONAL INFORMATION

U.S. Food and Drug Administration
www.fda.gov/cdrh/breastimplants/

Breast Augmentation & Breast
Implants Information
www.implantinfo.com

Cosmetic Surgery News
www.cosmeticsurgery-news.com

Cosmetic Surgery & Skin Care News
www.cosmetic-surgery-news.com

Male Aesthetic Surgery
By Daniel Marchac, Mark S. Granick,
Mark P. Solomon
A textbook, this is one of the few books that
covers cosmetic surgery for men.

**The Best Breast: The Ultimate,
Discriminating Woman's Guide to
Breast Augmentation**
By John B. Tebbetts, M.D.,
and Terrye B. Tebbetts

**Everything You Ever Wanted to
Know About Cosmetic Surgery But
Couldn't Afford to Ask**
By Alan Gaynor, M.D.

Chapter 8

What Is Liposuction?
Removing localized fat deposits 138

Liposuction for the Abdomen and Arms
Help for love handles and more 140 ·

The Tummy Tuck
Eliminating that bulging belly 142

Body Work

Recontouring the Upper Body
Smoothing out the back, breasts, neck, and more 144

Leaner Legs
A lift or lipo for the butt and hips on down 146

Building Up
Implants and more to add shape to calves and buttocks 148

Treating Leg Veins
Sclerotherapy for varicose and spider veins 150

Now What Do I Do?
Answers to common questions 152

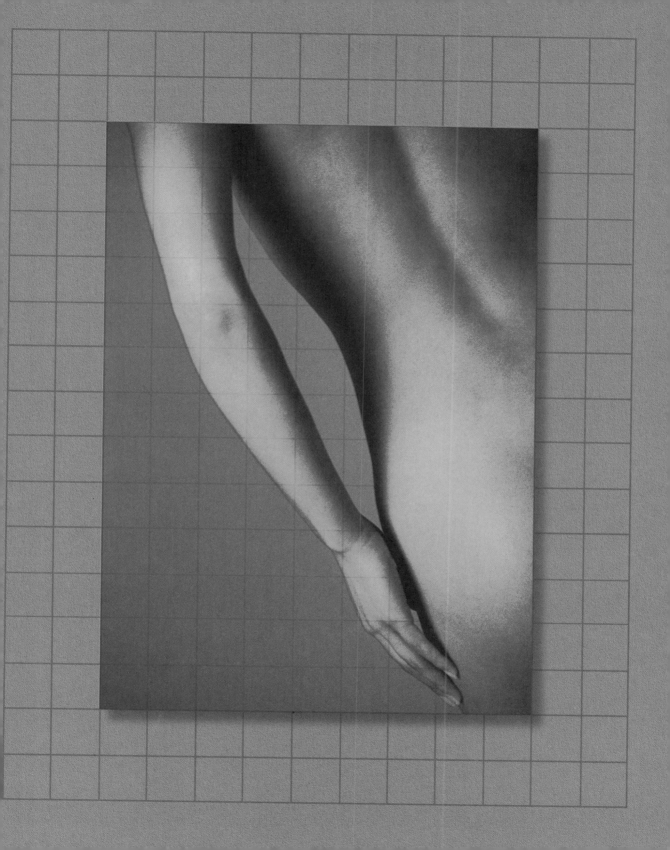

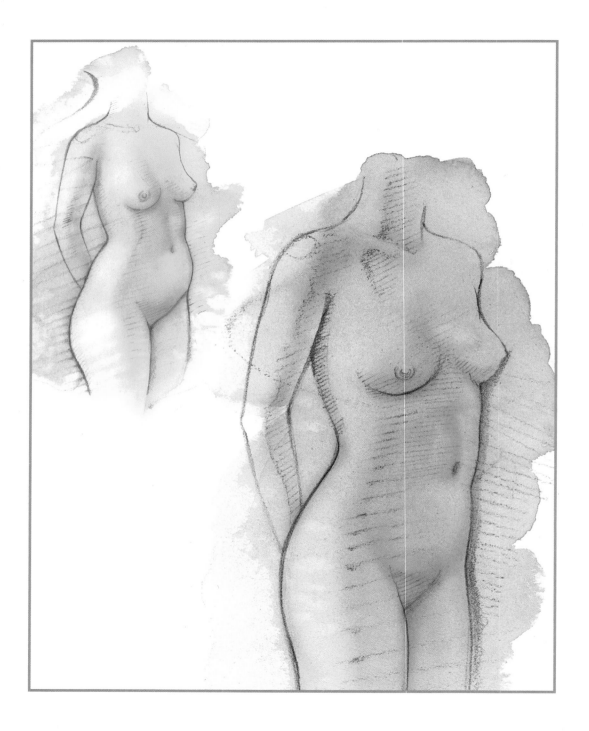

How much weight we gain is up to us; where it tends to accumulate on the body is dictated largely by heredity. The lucky ones are miracles of proportion; the unlucky have pockets of fat that no amount of diet and exercise can trim. Cosmetic surgeons have various techniques to contour the body into proportion, including adding shape and definition where it's lacking.

what is liposuction?

An overview of one of the most popular forms of cosmetic surgery

Liposuction (also known as **lipoplasty** and **liposculpture**) is the mechanical removal of localized fatty deposits that are resistant to diet and exercise. The key word here is *localized*. Lipo is most successful at removing isolated areas of fat—it is not a means of overall weight loss. The ideal candidate is a healthy person with good skin tone (elasticity) who is within 30% of his or her ideal weight. The procedure, using local or general anesthesia, can take anywhere from 30 minutes to a few hours, depending on how much fat is removed, how difficult the fat is to reach, and how many areas are being treated at one time.

Some newer techniques help break down the fat and make it easier to remove. In **tumescent**, or **superwet**, **lipoplasty**, large volumes of saline solution mixed with local anesthetic and adrenaline are injected into the fat to make the cells easier to remove. With **ultrasound-assisted lipoplasty** (UAL), sound waves break down and liquefy the fat cells before they are suctioned out. This technique is an effective addition to traditional lipo for removing fat from more fibrous areas, such as male breasts and love handles (fat pads at the side of the waist), and the upper back. Both variations have advantages and drawbacks, so be sure to discuss either thoroughly with your surgeon if he suggests it.

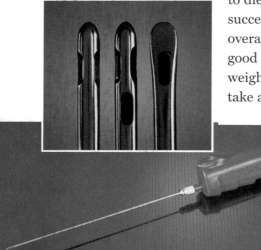

With traditional liposuction, the surgeon makes a tiny incision in the area to be treated and inserts a **cannula** (a thin, hollow metal rod, pictured) underneath the skin. The cannula is connected to a high-powered suction pump. The surgeon moves the cannula back and forth to dislodge and suction out the fat cells just beneath the skin.

ask the experts

What are the risks associated with liposuction?

You may experience infection or bleeding. The most common aesthetic risks are an uneven contour and skin surface irregularities, such as dents and dimpling. You could also have pigmentation changes, nerve damage, or fluid retention. Blood clots, excessive fluid loss (which could lead to shock), and perforation of organs, while rare, can also occur.

What is recovery like?

You'll have some swelling and bruising, and possibly numbness or a burning sensation at the treated areas. You might have to wear a compression garment regularly for 2 to 4 weeks to control swelling and shape your skin to its new contour. You will be able to return to work within a week and resume strenuous activity in less than a month. Complete healing occurs over time. Within 6 months the swelling will have subsided and you will have greater skin contraction.

What can I expect from this surgery?

You'll see a big change the day after surgery. A few weeks later you'll be even happier, and within 6 months you'll look even better. After lipo the skin will need to shrink to its new contour, and that takes time. In some cases lipo may need to be followed by a **lift** procedure to cut away excess skin because loose skin is not helped by liposuction.

How long will the results last?

The results should last a lifetime, but if you have significant weight gain later in life, you may need to have it redone.

FEES

Liposuction

Surgeons' fees are based on the site being treated. The more fat removed, and/or the more areas done, the bigger the fee. Liposuction of the neck can cost from $2,000 to $4,000; the arms from $3,000 to $5,000; the abdomen $3,000 to $6,000; thighs $4,000 to $7,000; and the knees, calves, and ankles from $4,000 to $6,000. Your surgeon may offer a discount if you're having more than one site done at a time.

liposuction for the abdomen and arms

What diet and exercise can't do for you, liposuction can

Liposuction is an ingenious solution to stubborn fatty deposits, especially in the upper arms and love handles. No amount of dieting or sit-ups can take off certain pockets of fat.

The area to be treated is first injected with a solution of anesthetic, **saline** (salt water), and **epinephrine** (to constrict blood vessels and reduce bleeding). Then your surgeon makes a very small hole—less than the width of a fingernail—hidden in a crease. Next, the doctor inserts beneath the skin a hollow metal rod that is connected to a high-powered suction pump, which sucks out the fat.

If you have a fleshy fullness underneath your upper arms (between the armpit and the elbow), you have a **batwing deformity**. In a relatively young person whose skin is still rather elastic, liposuction can address this. (For an older person, whose skin will not contract, the treatment option is **brachioplasty**, a procedure in which an incision is made from the elbow to the armpit, and excess fat, tissue, and skin are removed. Unfortunately, this surgery leaves a visible scar.)

Liposuction is not recommended for people with diabetes, heart or lung conditions, a history of blood clots, anemia, or poor skin tone (not enough elasticity). If you have had previous surgery in the same area, lipo may not be appropriate. Also, you must inform your surgeon if you have a hernia, which could be punctured during an abdominal procedure.

For lipo of the belly, the incision is often made near the belly button to camouflage the scar.

ask the experts

Is lipo a shortcut to weight loss?

Not at all. In fact, if you are very overweight, you will have to lose weight before you are a sound candidate for liposuction. This treatment is for the removal of small amounts of concentrated fat from individuals of normal weight.

My health spa now has a podiatrist on staff who can do liposuction for a lot less money than a plastic surgeon. Is this a good idea?

Not really. While liposuction has become an increasingly popular procedure, it is still a medical treatment and needs to be performed by a doctor who is certified, trained, and experienced in dealing with a variety of possible complications from liposuction.

FEES

Ab and Arm Liposuction

Surgeons' fees are based on the site being treated. The more fat removed, or the more areas done, the greater the fee. Liposuction of the arms ranges from $3,000 to $5,000; the abdomen $3,000 to $6,000. An arm lift runs from $3,000 to $8,000.

Is There a Cellulite Solution?

Cellulite, that lumpy fatty skin with a cottage cheese appearance, is a scourge to many women. It occurs mostly on the hips and thighs. While there is no permanent fix for this skin-texture problem, deep massage and various topical agents have been shown to temporarily diminish its appearance. This is also the case with the latest weapon in the war against such dimply skin, **Endermologie**, which is a high-tech machine (approved by the FDA) that applies a vacuum suction to the skin and underlying tissues. It requires ongoing treatments (monthly, if not more frequently)—which add up to real money—to maintain results. What causes cellulite? In certain fatty areas, you have extra fibrous bands of connective tissue that limit the tissue's ability to stretch, thereby giving your skin a dimpled look. It affects mostly women (few young girls or men have it). It appears to be somewhat genetic and to happen with age. Weight loss and exercise are the two best means of fighting cellulite, but you may not be able to get rid of it.

the tummy tuck

When you need surgery to eliminate that bulging belly

If your problem is a bulge or sagging created by loose skin, then liposuction is not the answer. Instead, that skin needs to be cut away. Loose abdominal skin is a common byproduct of pregnancy, large weight loss, or naturally weak abdominal muscles.

To reduce the abdomen, a plastic surgeon can perform an **abdominoplasty**, otherwise known as the **tummy tuck**. There are several variations of the tummy tuck, from mini to modified to full. Typically, with any of the tuck procedures, your surgeon will use liposuction to remove fat along with tightening, or repairing, the weakened underlying muscles of the abdomen, and removing excess or sagging skin. From a mini to a modified to a full tuck, more muscle is tightened and more skin is cut away.

With the mini tuck, your surgeon is making a small incision in the pubic hairline (it looks like a C-section scar), going from there to the belly button. With the modified, using a larger incision, he's taking out a little more skin and tightening the muscles a few inches above the belly button. The incision for the full tummy tuck is like a smile that goes from hipbone to hipbone along the pubic hairline. More skin is cut away and the muscles are tightened with permanent sutures all the way from the pubic bone up to the chest bone, which flattens a bulging belly.

Note: A mini tuck is often the fix for those with a pouching belly, which is caused by a common separation of the paired rectus muscles in the abdomen. Lipo cannot address this because tightening, not suction, is needed to close the muscle in order to flatten it. Sit-ups won't help either, because they strengthen the muscle but don't close it.

@sk the experts

What are the risks associated with a tuck procedure?

As with all forms of surgery, you risk infection, scarring, or **hematoma** (a collection of blood). (For risks associated with liposuction, see page 139).

What is recovery like and how long should the results last?

Incisional procedures, such as a tummy tuck, are more invasive than liposuction and therefore require slightly more recovery time. You may have to wear a compression garment for 2 or more weeks, and it may take a month before you are able to return to work. (See page 139 for more information on recovery from liposuction.) The results should last a lifetime, but if you have significant weight gain later, you may need to have it redone.

Can lipo or a tummy tuck give me six-pack abs?

No. Liposuction will reduce the fat layer over the muscle, but then you need to exercise. Beware of a fairly new and controversial lipo technique called **abdominal etching**, which contours the stomach area to create a more defined, muscular appearance. This treatment presents greater risks.

When Lipo Isn't the Answer

Liposuction represents the ultimate in minimally invasive body surgery. A plastic surgeon will always try to avoid cutting on the body—whether it's the arms, the thighs, the abdomen—because scars here are much more conspicuous than those associated with a facelift, where the incisions are hidden around the ear and in the hairline. However, if you have bulges and sags created by loose skin, liposuction is not the fix. Instead, you'll need to undergo an excisional procedure, such as a lift, to cut away the loose skin.

recontouring the upper body

Reducing the back, breasts, neck, and more

Usually when you think of liposuction, the first thing that comes to mind is reducing the thighs, tummy, or buttocks. But it can do much more, improving the upper arms, parts of the face and other areas. Liposuction is, after all, the primary method of body contouring. But when the skin is loose, you must turn to **lift procedures**, which involve cutting out skin to pull it taut and smooth it out.

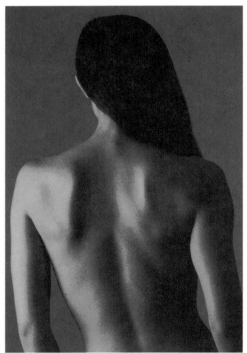

For example, if you are a 20-year-old woman and have a 50-year-old mother, and you both have a double chin, as a 20-year-old you will be a good candidate for liposuction of the neck. Your surgeon will be able to successfully remove the fat and your skin will contract because it is youthful and elastic. For your mother, lipo will need to be followed by a lift because her older skin will not recoil enough to achieve the desired result, and the lipo could then make the skin look even looser. (Liposuction can also reduce the fat in the cheeks and jowls. For more information on contouring the cheeks, chin, jowls, and neck, see pages 166 to 173.)

A flabby back can be smoothed through liposuction of the rolls that may appear below the shoulder blades. If you have too much loose skin there, it will need to be cut away.

ask the experts

Can liposuction be used for a breast or chest reduction?

Only a small percentage of women and men can have liposuction to successfully reduce the breast or chest area. What determines the treatment option is the percentage of fat in the breast, how loose the breast skin is, and how much the nipple sags. For more on breast and chest reduction, see pages 124 and 130.

What are the risks associated with these procedures?

There is a risk of infection, severe scarring or **hematoma** (a pool of blood under the skin). With liposuction, there is also a risk of **asymmetry** (unevenness in an area) and skin surface irregularities, such as rippling and dimpling. You could also experience pigmentation changes or fluid retention. Though rare, excessive fluid loss, which could lead to shock, may occur.

How long will the results last?

Most body contouring procedures are one-time operations. Although you might want to repeat a procedure later in life should you gain weight, the expectation is to do it once and then stick to a sensible diet and exercise.

FEES

Reducing Above the Waist

Surgeons' fees are typically by the site, and whether you will be having more than one site worked on during the same procedure. Liposuction of the neck can cost from $2,000 to $4,000, and the arms from $3,000 to $5,000.

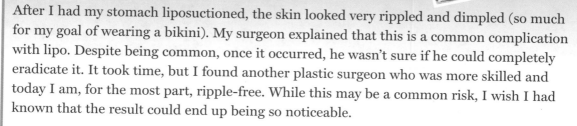

CAUTIONARY TALE

The not-so-flat belly

After I had my stomach liposuctioned, the skin looked very rippled and dimpled (so much for my goal of wearing a bikini). My surgeon explained that this is a common complication with lipo. Despite being common, once it occurred, he wasn't sure if he could completely eradicate it. It took time, but I found another plastic surgeon who was more skilled and today I am, for the most part, ripple-free. While this may be a common risk, I wish I had known that the result could end up being so noticeable.

Beth F., Northampton, Massachusetts

leaner legs

Spot reduction from the butt and hips to the ankles

While liposuction can be used to reduce pockets of fat on your inner and outer thighs and buttocks, it can't tighten sagging skin and firm up tissue. To get a lean-looking leg, you need a **lift procedure**. This involves cutting out a wedge of skin and underlying fat. This surgery takes from 1 to $3\frac{1}{2}$ hours, using general anesthesia.

For the thighs and buttocks, your surgeon will perform either an **inner-thigh lift** or an **outer-thigh lift**. He makes an incision on both sides at the waistline, continuing around to the back, and removes a wedge of skin and fat. The incision for the **hip lift** is smaller. The incisions should be positioned so the scars will be covered by underwear or a bathing suit. With the thigh lifts, the incision wraps around the upper leg. The scar will be noticeable and permanent, though it should fade over time. The incision can sometimes be made inside the natural crease where the buttocks meet the thigh, but this technique reduces the amount of skin and fat that can be removed.

Because the ankles, calves, and inner knees offer no place to hide a scar, excisional (cutting) procedures are rarely performed on these areas. Fortunately, liposuction, with its small incision and minimal invasiveness, can be used to sculpt these areas.

Do you need to wear a compression garment after undergoing a body contouring procedure? Visit one of these online stores for suitable items:

www.contemporarydesigninc.com
www.carrothersltd.com

ask the experts

Why can't all the fat be liposuctioned out of my thighs?

The more fat that is removed from a body part, the more loose and saggy the skin covering it becomes. If you were to have too much fat suctioned from your thighs, you'd be left with unattractive folds of loose flesh, which would then have to be cut off.

What are the risks associated with these procedures?

Infection, severe scarring, or **hematoma** (a collection of blood under the skin) may occur. With liposuction, you may experience **asymmetry**, or unevenness in an area. A complication common with lipo is skin irregularities, including rippling and dimpling. You could also have pigmentation changes or fluid retention.

What happens after the surgery? What is recovery like?

After liposuction, you'll have some swelling and bruising, along with numbness or burning. You will be able to return to work within a week or so, and resume strenuous activity in about a month. By 6 months the swelling will have subsided substantially. After lipo or a lifting procedure, it will be difficult to sit for several days. With a lift, it will be 2 weeks before you can return to work, and you will have to refrain from strenuous activity for 2 months.

How long will the results last?

Most body contouring procedures are one-time operations. Although you might want to repeat a procedure later in life should you gain weight, the expectation is to do it once, then follow a sensible diet and exercise.

FEES

Reducing Below the Waist

Surgeons' fees are typically by the site, and vary depending on whether you will be having more than one site worked on during the same operation. Liposuction of the thighs can cost from $4,000 to $7,000; for the knees, calves, and ankles $4,000 to $6,000. An outer-thigh lift (inclusive of the buttocks or hips) runs from $4,000 to $12,000; an inner-thigh lift from $3,000 to $10,000.

building up

Adding shape and definition to your calves and buttocks

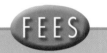

Calf and Buttocks Implants

Surgeons' fees for calf augmentation of both legs range from $3,000 to $6,000. This procedure is not covered by insurance unless it is deemed medically necessary for victims of polio or other degenerative muscular diseases or an accident that requires reconstruction. Buttock augmentation ranges from $3,000 to $6,000, depending on the technique used.

Some people can do calf exercises until the cows come home and never develop the muscle definition they desire. Others may just be self-conscious about their lack of a gentle curve. Regardless of the reason for your dissatisfaction, a **calf augmentation** (implant) may be for you.

For this procedure, your surgeon makes an incision behind the knee. He creates a small pocket in the calf on top of the muscle and beneath the **fascia** (the dense layer of connective tissue between the muscle and the skin). Next, your surgeon slides the solid silicone implant into the space, resting it on top of the muscle. The pocket must be large enough to accommodate the implant but snug enough so that the implant can't slide around. This 2-hour procedure can be done using local or general anesthesia, in an outpatient facility or a hospital.

If you're unhappy with your very flat seat, you may want to undergo a **buttock augmentation**. This can be achieved through one of three means: fat injection (using your own fat that has been liposuctioned from elsewhere on your body), **dermal grafts** (using tissue taken from another part of your body), or silicone implants (similar to calf implants).

Silicone calf and buttock implants may last a lifetime unless something causes them to shift. However, a large weight gain could undo the success of either procedure. If you use fat injections in the buttocks, you may need to repeat the procedure from two months to two years later, because the body absorbs recycled fat. Dermal grafts vary in how long they last, though with a new micro-grafting technique 50% to 75% of the fat grafted appears to survive long term.

ask the experts

What risks are associated with these procedures?

Asymmetry (uneven calves or buttocks) is a risk, as is the shifting of the implant in the pocket. Because the area into which the calf implant is inserted is a tight space, the implant could compress the muscle, compromise the blood supply, and cause tissue loss. Poor scarring can also result with either implant, despite the incision being made behind the knee for the calf surgery to minimize its appearance.

What happens after the surgery? What is recovery like?

The biggest issue for any lower-extremity procedure is swelling. With a calf implant, you will be significantly swollen for 4 to 6 weeks, and moderately swollen for the next 6 to 12 months. You will be able to walk right away, but must avoid strenuous activity for a month. And your legs must be elevated whenever you're not walking (put your feet up at work, in bed). Also, for several weeks you will not be able to travel by plane due to the risk of swelling. Your doctor may request that you wear a compression garment (see page 146), tape, or dressing on the leg. No matter which option is used, you'll have to make sure no pressure is put on the calf, which could injure the muscle beneath the implant. The discomfort caused by buttock implants will put you out of commission for several days to a week. Fat injections or grafts will cause only mild discomfort, though you will need to wear a compression garment for up to 6 weeks.

How safe is the silicone implant itself?

The silicone implant used here is made from a stable, solid block, so there is nothing to leak. (For more on silicone and safety, see page 120.)

Why might I be a poor candidate for a calf implant?

If your legs are amorphous due to obesity, or you are a smoker, a calf implant is probably not for you. In either case, blood flow to the skin may be compromised and tissue loss could occur.

treating leg veins

Eliminating varicose and spider veins

They are called spider veins—thin red veins in the legs. Their medical name is **sunburst varicosities**. They are often accompanied by painful **varicose veins** (larger blue and sometimes bulging veins). Both can be treated with cosmetic surgery.

For varicose veins, **sclerotherapy** is the best fix. Here, a chemical solution is injected into the unwanted vein, irritating the vessel wall. The sclerosing, or hardening, of the vessel closes it down and destroys it. The body absorbs the vessel, so it fades from view. Varicose veins are already damaged and poorly functioning, so they can be eliminated without posing a circulatory problem because nearby healthy veins take up the rerouted blood flow.

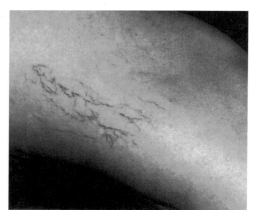

Unsightly spider veins can be erased with sclerotherapy.

Before the procedure, you may be tested to make sure you have enough competent veins in your legs. If not, you may need to have a small surgical procedure to fix some of the vessels before getting the injections. (Faulty vessels, or valves, are due to the weakening of the vein walls, chiefly from pregnancy and other hormonal changes, as well as from prolonged standing, obesity, and genetics.)

For spider veins, or for those who are extremely needle-phobic, lasers are the alternative. Lasers are also very good at treating resistant small leg veins. Laser treatment is actually more uncomfortable than sclerotherapy, however. Laser energy heats up the blood vessels in order to shrink or destroy them.

ask the experts

What are the risks involved with these procedures?

Bruising is common. There's a chance that new blood vessels will surface. There's also the possibility of **hyperpigmentation**, a dark spot forming where a blood vessel has been removed, which can take months to go away. You could experience **matting**, which is the appearance of many fine blood vessels in the area where larger blood vessels have been destroyed. (Lasers are usually more effective than injections in treating this complication.) With injections, complications are uncommon, but blood clots, ulcers, or **phlebitis**, which is an inflammation of the blood vessel, can occur. There are rare reports of allergic reactions to some of the solutions.

What happens after the treatment? What is recovery like?

After injections or laser treatments, you will need to wear compression hose or bandages for 2 to 7 days, depending on the size of the vessels treated. You can go back to work immediately. While you should avoid strenuous exercise for 2 days, walking is fine. You should see improvement within 2 to 8 weeks.

How many sessions will I need?

Whether you're having sclerotherapy or laser treatment, it usually takes 5 to 8 sessions of 15 to 60 minutes each. In a single sclerotherapy session, numerous relatively painless injections are given, with each covering about an inch of vein. Sometimes you can't get rid of all visible blood vessels, but you should see a considerable reduction. If you have very large varicose veins, you may need a vascular surgeon to surgically tie off or remove the blood vessels.

What can I do about the noticeable veins on my back?

Sclerotherapy can be used for blood vessels on the belly, breasts, back and face. Laser treatment is also successful. (See page 50 for information on lasers.)

FEES

Vein Reduction

Doctors' fees for sclerotherapy injections range from $200 to $500 per session, based on the amount of the solution injected. Laser therapy costs between $350 and $650 per session. Though this is usually an elective procedure and not covered by insurance, if your varicose veins are being treated for medical reasons, such as painful throbbing or swelling, your insurance may cover part of the cost.

now what do I do?

Answers to common questions

Once I've had liposuction, will the fat come back, either in the same place or elsewhere?

No. The reason people sometimes think they've gained fat in another area after having had the procedure is because the site that was liposuctioned had previously served as a barometer: When they gained weight, they gained it there. Lipo brings more proportion to weight distribution, so if you gain pounds after the procedure it appears to have "gone elsewhere." For example, if you had lipo done on your hips and then gained weight, the new weight will go to both your hips and your belly, whereas before it would have all gone to your hips.

Can liposuction get rid of my cellulite?

Cellulite, which is lumpy fatty skin with a cottage cheese appearance, is not improved by liposuction because this treatment is not fixing skin, it's removing fat. See page 141 for more on cellulite.

Can liposuction remove all my fat in any given area?

No, and here's why: Fat exists in many layers in the body. Liposuction can remove the fat that is just below the skin, but not the fat that is inside the muscle and deeper.

Can the fat liposuctioned from my buttocks be used elsewhere in my body?

Fat from your buttocks or any other part of your body can be transferred to your aging, wrinkled hands or creases in your face to plump up those areas. Along with smoothing out lines, this harvested fat can also be used to fill in cheek hollows or other contour defects. But because the body absorbs recycled fat, it's hard to know how long it will last.

Can fat removal make me healthier by, say, lowering my risk of heart disease?

Not if you have a beer belly, meaning you have fat above and below the muscle. Liposuction can only take out the fat that is just below the skin, but it's fat that sits below the muscle and surrounds the organs (known as **intra-abdominal,** or **apple, fat**), that is associated with heart disease. Women are increasingly at risk for heart disease after menopause, when they tend to develop a belly, whereas men are at risk at a younger age because they always have a tendency to accumulate fat there.

How old is too old or how young too young for liposuction?

A person of almost any age who is in good health, has good skin tone, and is of normal weight is a candidate for liposuction. If you are older and your skin is less elastic, you may need surgery to cut away excess skin in addition to or instead of liposuction.

Now where do I go?!

CONTACTS	ADDITIONAL INFORMATION
American Society of Plastic Surgeons **www.plasticsurgery.org** 847-228-9900	U.S. Food and Drug Administration **www.fda.gov**
American Society for Aesthetic Plastic Surgery **www.surgery.org** 212-921-0500	Cosmetic Surgery News **www.cosmeticsurgery-news.com** Cosmetic Surgery & Skin Care News **www.cosmetic-surgery-news.com**
American Academy of Facial Plastic and Reconstructive Surgery **www.aafprs.org** 800-332-FACE	

Chapter 9

Smoothing the Forehead
What a forehead lift can do for you   158

Eyes Revised
Eliminating puffiness and more   160

Fixing the Ears
Help for protruding ears and hanging lobes   162

Lip Service
How to plump up or reduce the lips 164

Parts of the Face

Cheek Chic
For a leaner, more angular look 166

Jowl Reduction
Put an end to jiggling jowls 168

Chin Up
Receding or jutting out—surgery to improve your profile   170

Neck Lifts
For a more graceful-looking neckline 172

Now What Do I Do?
Answers to common questions 174

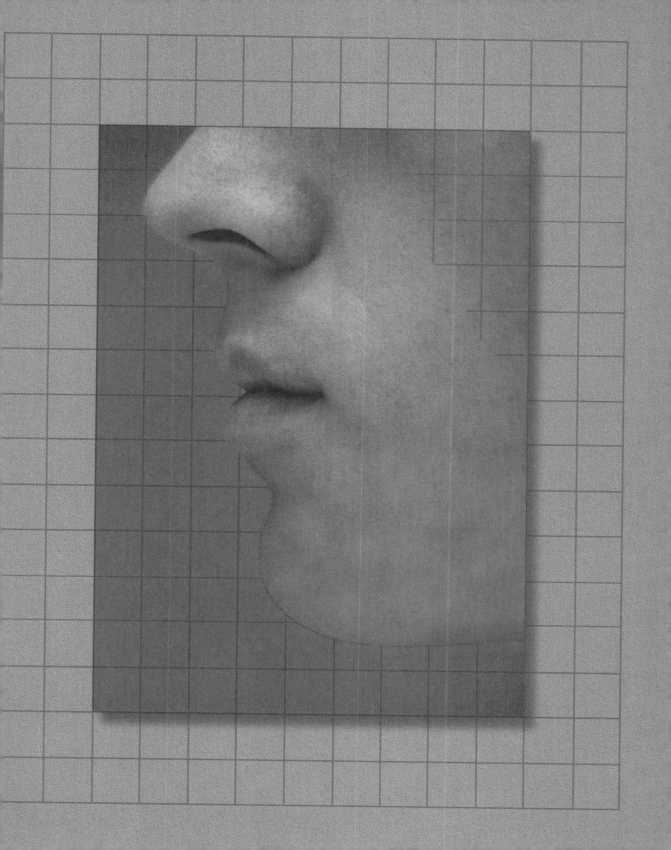

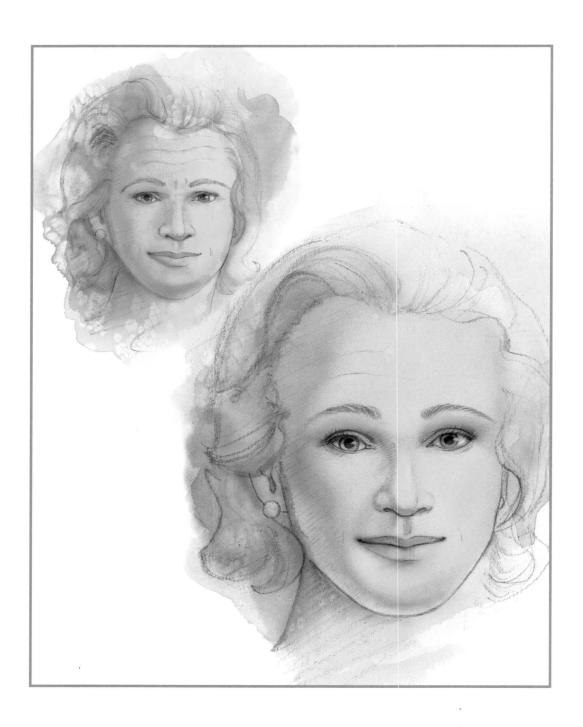

When you look in the mirror, what do you see? Maybe you have always disliked a particular feature, such as a weak chin. Or maybe you are just beginning to notice the toll time and gravity are taking—crow's feet around the eyes, sagging jowls. Plastic surgery can improve not only your aging appearance but also your outlook.

smoothing the forehead

Ease those frown lines and that wrinkled brow

After age 40 telltale signs of aging begin to appear on the forehead: deepening vertical creases between your eyes (frown lines), horizontal wrinkles that run across the top of your forehead (a furrowed brow), and a general sagging of the brow (which may make you look perpetually tired or sad). The skin above the eyes may also begin to droop, causing them to appear hooded.

If your main concern is wrinkles and lines on your forehead, injections of **Botox** (a substance that relaxes muscles) will flatten them out, but this is a temporary fix that requires ongoing maintenance. (For more on Botox, see page 34.) If lines are a problem along with sagging or drooping skin, the solution is a **forehead lift**, also known as a **brow lift.** This can be performed under local or general anesthesia and is typically an outpatient procedure that takes from 1 to 2 hours, depending on which technique is used and the extent of the area being worked on.

There are a few variations in technique. The traditional **coronal lift** method calls for your surgeon to make an incision from ear to ear across the top of your scalp within the hairline. The forehead skin is then lifted up and the excess tissue and any muscle that is causing the lines are removed or altered.

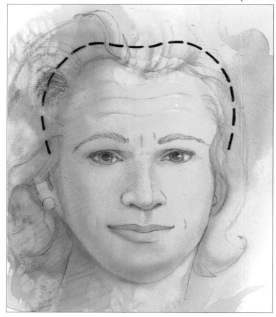

Because the traditional incision is made in the scalp, the scars will not be visible, but your hairline will be raised and you run a risk of hair loss.

ask the experts

What if I don't want a big incision on top of my head?

In addition to the coronal lift, there are two other places your surgeon can make the incision. With the **anterior hairline lift**, which raises the brows without raising the hairline, the cut is made along the frontal hairline. Although the scar should eventually fade to a fine line, you may need to comb your hair forward to cover it. An **endoscopic lift** involves just 3 or more short incisions in the hairline and a tiny camera inserted through one of the incisions to guide the surgeon beneath the skin. This procedure eliminates the large ear-to-ear incision but has limitations.

What if only the corners of my eyebrows droop?

You can have a **temporal lift**. This is essentially one third of a brow lift, which raises both the inner and outer parts. The temporal procedure will just lift the outer edges of the brow.

What are the risks associated with a brow lift?

Among the most common are infection and **hematoma** (a pooling of blood under the skin). The incision may be itchy and numb for weeks or even months. With incisions made in the hair you may have permanent hair loss. Scarring is possible, as is nerve damage, which could result in muscle weakness, loss of motion, or **asymmetry** (an uneven appearance).

What is recovery like?

You may have headaches. The incision area will be bruised and swollen for about 2 weeks, and you may experience swelling and bruising around the cheeks and eyes for several days. You'll be able to return to work in 5 to 10 days. You can wear makeup and wash and color your hair in 2 to 5 days, but you won't be able to wear contact lenses for a week. Strenuous activity can be resumed in a few weeks, but you'll have to avoid direct sun exposure for several months.

FEES

Brow Lift

Surgeons' fees range from $2,500 to $6,500, depending on which technique you have and the extent of the area being treated. This is an elective procedure and therefore not covered by insurance unless you have such extreme sagging of the forehead or brows that it interferes with your vision.

eyes revised

Eyelid surgery can help put the sparkle back

Because of the thinness of the skin around the eyes, this area is one of the first to show signs of aging. That's why the eyelid surgery called **blepharoplasty** is among the most frequently performed cosmetic procedures. Depending on your problem, your surgeon can treat just the upper or lower eyelids, or both at the same time. With lower lid blepharoplasty, fine lines and puffiness below the eyes are minimized by removing (or redistributing) excess fatty tissue, skin, and muscle. This is traditionally done with a scalpel through an incision made just below the lower eyelashes. Another option for the lower lid only is a **transconjunctival blepharoplasty**, where the incision is made on the inside of the eyelid so there is no external scarring. With this method, however, only fatty bulges, not excess skin, can be removed.

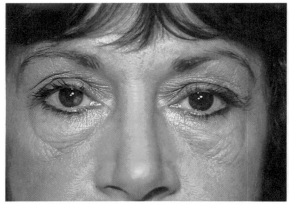 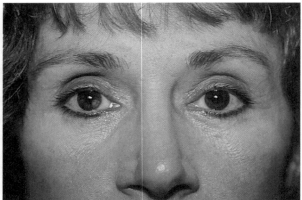

Patient photographs of blepharoplasty courtesy of Dr. Stephen Perkins, AAFPRS

To combat excessive wrinkles and sagging skin in and around the upper lid, the plastic surgeon makes an incision in the natural fold of the upper eyelid. Then the excess tissue and skin are removed with a scalpel or laser. If a laser is used, you'll have to wear protective covers or special contacts to protect your eyes.

ask the experts

What can't eyelid surgery fix?

Crow's feet, which are lines at the sides of your eyes, should be treated with **Botox** injections (see page 34) or skin-resurfacing procedures (see page 54). Undereye circles are improved with bleaching agents and skin resurfacing, and sagging eyebrows are fixed with a **brow lift** (see page 158).

What are the risks associated with eyelid surgery?

The main risks are bleeding and infection. If too much skin is removed from the upper lid, you may have difficulty closing your eye; if too much is removed from the lower lid, **eversion** (a turning down of the lid) may occur. Removing too much fat will result in a gaunt look. Your eyelids could become scarred or heal unevenly. You may temporarily experience dryness, burning, itching, or excessive tearing. You can become sensitive to light for a few weeks, or have blurred or double vision. Blindness, while extremely rare, can occur.

What happens after the surgery? What is recovery like?

The bruising and swelling you'll experience in the first several weeks can be alleviated by applying ice packs and keeping your head elevated. During that time, swelling may hinder your ability to completely close your eyes. Until this subsides you should lubricate your eyes before going to sleep with an ophthalmic ointment and eyedrops. You won't be able to wear contact lenses for several days to several weeks after surgery, and you may have difficulty reading or watching TV for 2 or 3 days. After 3 to 5 days, your stitches will be taken out. You can go back to work in 5 to 10 days, but must refrain from strenuous activity or any heavy exertion (even bending over, sex, or having a heated argument) for nearly 3 weeks. You'll need to wear sunblock and sunglasses when you go out in the sun. The results should last about 10 years.

FEES

Blepharoplasty

Surgeons' fees range from $2,000 to $3,500 for upper or lower eyelids, and from $3,000 to $7,000 for both. (If you are considering both, it may be less expensive to do them together.) While this elective procedure is usually not covered by insurance, upper-eyelid surgery may be covered, at least in part, if it is necessary to improve your field of vision.

fixing the ears

Help for protruding ears and hanging lobes

If the size or shape of your ears has you feeling self-conscious, consider **otoplasty**, which is surgery to reshape the cartilage and thus reposition, flatten, or reduce the size of the ears.

Otoplasty is most commonly done to pin back ears that stick out. Because ears are almost fully formed by the age of 5, this procedure is often performed on children. During the surgery, which lasts between $1^1/_2$ and 3 hours for both ears, your surgeon will remove or reshape a portion of cartilage from the back of the ear and use permanent sutures to make the ear lie flatter. The surgery can be performed using local or general anesthesia and is usually done on an outpatient basis.

Have you considered that even your earlobes can begin to show your age as the skin sags, making the lobes appear long and pendulous? With an **earlobe reduction**, which is often done along with a facelift, your surgeon can remove part of the lobe to shorten it. This procedure, using local or general anesthesia (depending on whether it's done with the facelift), takes about a half hour to do both earlobes.

Patient photographs of otoplasty
courtesy of R. Gregory Smith, M.D., Ponte Vedra, FL

@sk the experts

Will my pinned-back ears stay that way?

While the results should be permanent, the problem can recur. Typically ears stick out if there is too much cartilage in one part of the ear and cartilage in another area that isn't sufficiently curled back. Because you're working against the forces of the cartilage, there is a chance it could give way and snap back into its original position. This is more likely to happen if the surgery is done as an adult, when the cartilage is firmer and more difficult to remold. If it does, the procedure can be repeated.

What risks are involved with ear procedures?

While your hearing should be unaffected, bleeding and infection can occur. You may have some numbness and scarring. A blood clot may form on the ear and need to be drained. You could end up with mismatched or artificial-looking ears—though it should be noted that no one is born with perfectly matched ears.

What is recovery like?

You'll wear a bandage for 2 to 5 days to help with the reshaping, possibly followed by an elastic headband for 4 to 6 weeks. Your ears will be swollen and may ache, throb, or look red. The stitches will be removed in 8 or 9 days. You will not be able to sleep on your side for a few days. You can return to work or school in about a week and resume your normal routine in about 10 to 14 days. Strenuous activity and contact sports should be halted for 4 to 8 weeks. It may take several weeks for the swelling to subside enough for you to see the final outcome.

FEES

Ear Surgery

Surgeons' fees for pinning the ears back range from $2,500 to $8,500 for both ears—less if only one ear is treated. An earlobe reduction runs between $750 and $900 per ear. While ear surgery is an elective procedure, if your condition is due to improper development or injury it may be covered, at least in part, by your insurance provider.

lip service

Kiss your too-thin grin good-bye

Lip enhancement surgery can do wondrous things. A **lip augmentation** can give an overall boost to thin lips. A **lip lift** can plump up an upper lip that has thinned and drooped with age. And a **lip reduction** can reduce the size of your lips. No matter which procedure you're considering, bear in mind that you can only enhance what you were born with—not change the intrinsic shape of your lips. Each procedure takes about an hour and can be done using local or general anesthesia.

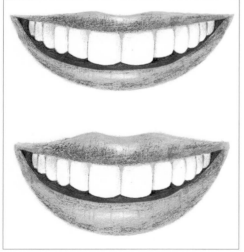

Injectables and implants can increase the volume of aging or inadequate lips. They can also add crispness and definition to the edges.

Think of your lip as a sausage casing that, with augmentation, your dermatologist or plastic surgeon can plump up by filling with a substance—commonly collagen (see page 36) or fat taken from elsewhere on your body (see page 38). Either of these injectable materials offers only a temporary enlargement—the procedure must be repeated to maintain results. Implants can also be inserted in a surgical procedure. They are made of sheets of donor tissue and other synthetic materials.

A lip lift can be done in one of three ways: by making an incision in the natural crease beneath the nostrils and pulling up on the lip; by making an incision where the vermillion (the pink lip skin) meets the outer skin and lifting the lip (called a **lip advancement**); or by cinching (suturing) the tissue on the inside of the upper lip.

In a lip reduction, your surgeon will remove a strip of tissue ($\frac{1}{4}$- to $\frac{1}{2}$-inch) from inside the lip, which will pull the lip down and in.

@sk the experts

What risks are associated with lip procedures?

Numbness, infection, and scarring may occur, though any numbness should be temporary. If you have a substance injected into your lips, it can become unevenly absorbed by the surrounding tissue. An implant can extrude (your body can push it out of your lip), or gradually become absorbed or shrink and need to be replaced.

What is recovery like?

If a lip augmentation is done with injectable material, recovery time is minimal. For all other procedures, you will be swollen and bruised for 3 days to a week and must be careful not to bump or jar your lips. In addition, eating and brushing your teeth may be a bit uncomfortable for a couple of days. For the first few days following surgery, you can reduce the swelling and discomfort by applying cold compresses and keeping your head elevated. After 4 or 5 days you can resume wearing lipstick, but be careful not to rub it off. You can return to work within a week.

How long will the results from my lip surgery last?

The results with a lift, implant, or reduction should be long lasting. Augmentation achieved with injections will only be temporary and will require ongoing treatment.

FEES

Lip Treatment

Surgeons' fees for procedures to lift or reduce the lips range from $1,500 to $2,000. Implants for enlarging the lips cost from $1,000 to $3,000. Injectables range from $250 to $500 or more per session, depending on the substance you have injected (a fat transfer is higher). Also, because injectable material dissipates over time, the treatment will have to be repeated periodically—usually in a few months—so you must factor in the cost of ongoing treatment.

cheek chic

Create the contour you desire

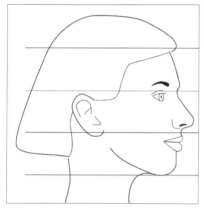

Ideally, the three parts of the face—the brow, the nose, and the chin area—are in proportion. Cheek implants can help restore balance to the face.

Altering the shape of the cheeks can have a significant impact on the face, especially if the cheeks are sunken or poorly defined. To improve cheekbone structure, a plastic surgeon can perform a **malar augmentation**, or cheek enhancement surgery. With this procedure, implants made of synthetic material are inserted behind the facial muscles to build up and support sagging tissue. To eliminate external scarring, the implants can be inserted through an incision in the mouth.

An alternative to implants is the repositioning of fat in your face to create higher, more prominent cheekbones. Here, the fat that has sagged into your jowls is pulled back up over the cheekbones (similar to a facelift; see page 182). This is done two ways: by undercutting the fat and lifting it, or by folding the fat back up to where it came from and stitching it in place. Still another option is to remove some of the fat right below the cheek.

At the other extreme, if you think your cheeks are too chubby or you simply want a more angular appearance, your surgeon can remove the **buccal fat pad**. This fatty tissue, about the size of a large marble in an adult, lies just below the cheek area. It can be removed through an incision made inside your mouth, near the molars, so there is no visible scarring.

Each of these procedures is typically done on an outpatient basis, using local or general anesthesia. They take 30 minutes to 2 hours, depending on the technique used and the extent of the area being treated.

FEES

Cheek Surgery

Surgeons' fees range from $2,500 to $6,000, depending on the technique used.

ask the experts

What are the risks associated with these procedures?

Cheek implants can shift or be improperly positioned, causing **asymmetry** (uneven cheeks). Bleeding can occur. If the area treated becomes infected, the implant may have to be removed. **Capsular contracture**, a hardening of scar tissue around the implant, could occur, resulting in an unnatural look. Nerve damage, while rare, is a possibility.

What is recovery like?

If you get implants, it will take 2 weeks or so for the swelling and bruising to diminish. Applying cold compresses and keeping your head elevated can help. If the incision is made inside your mouth, you may have to go on a liquid or soft food diet for the first few days following surgery to keep food particles from the incision; chewing may be limited for several days. You'll also have to avoid using a toothbrush near the incision until it's healed. Most of the swelling will subside in 2 to 4 weeks, but you will need to guard against bumping or jarring your face for at least 6 weeks. The results may not be apparent until all the swelling has subsided (usually in about 3 or 4 months), but they should be permanent. With the buccal fat pad removal you can return to work immediately.

jowl reduction

Get rid of sagging jowls

The jowls, the area below the cheeks, tend to droop and sag with age. Fortunately, there are several different cosmetic surgery remedies: a **facelift** (see page 180), a **neck lift** (see page 172), **cheek enhancement** (see page 166), and **liposuction** (see page 138).

Work on the jowl area requires, for the most part, the removal of fat. For this to be effective, the skin around your jowls has to be elastic enough to contract back to a new, sleeker jawline. If it can't, the only option is a facelift, where the excess skin can be tightened. To remove the fat, a plastic surgeon will use liposuction, a procedure that suctions out fat below the skin. Here, an incision is made behind the ear, then the fat in the jowl is vacuumed out. Often, liposuction is combined with the removal of the **buccal fat pad**, the marble-sized fatty tissue that lies just below each cheekbone. The buccal fat pads will be removed through incisions inside the mouth, near the molars. This dual procedure will create a more defined and angular cheek and jaw. The surgery is usually performed in an outpatient setting, using local or general anesthesia.

ask the experts

What are the risks associated with these procedures?

As with any surgery, bleeding or infection can occur. While you can take out less of the buccal fat pad, you can't take more if you've removed it entirely and you're unhappy after the procedure. Liposuction risks include **asymmetry** (uneven sides), rippling and dimpling in the skin, pigmentation changes, and fluid retention.

What is recovery like?

You may be swollen or bruised for a few days following liposuction. You'll have to take extra care when chewing or brushing your teeth to ensure that you don't disturb the incision. Most of the noticeable swelling will subside in 2 to 4 weeks, but you'll need to guard against bumping your face for at least 6 weeks. You may experience numbness and a burning sensation in the affected area. Complete healing will occur gradually, but by 6 months the swelling will have subsided substantially. The results should be long lasting.

Jowl Reduction

Surgeons' fees vary depending on the technique used and the extent of the area being treated. Using liposuction, your doctor will typically work on both the jowl and the neck, which runs about $3,000 to $4,000.

chin up
Improve your profile

If your weak chin or jutting jaw is spoiling your looks, **mentoplasty** (also called **genioplasty**) can bring proportion to a profile by building up, reducing, or reshaping the chin.

Enlarging the chin (known as **chin augmentation**) is accomplished either with the insertion of an implant (usually made of solid silicone, Teflon, or Dacron) or by moving the bone forward (see jaw restructuring on page 110). If an implant is being used, traditionally your surgeon will make an incision in the natural crease underneath the chin, where the scar will be less visible. Using a different technique the incision is made inside your mouth in the groove between the teeth and lower lip, thereby leaving no external scar. For either method, your surgeon will separate all of the tissue from the jawbone to create a pocket for the implant. Once the implant is inserted, the incision is closed. Best of all, the jaw doesn't have to be wired shut during recovery—as it often does when surgery involves repositioning the bone or the entire lower jaw.

In the case of chin reduction, an incision is also made inside the mouth or under the chin, and the jawbone is resculpted.

Chin surgery can take from 30 minutes to 3 hours, depending on the procedure and the extent of the work, and is performed in an outpatient setting, using local or general anesthesia. It can be performed on teenagers and adults.

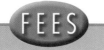

FEES

Chin Surgery

Surgeons' fees range from $2,000 to $6,000, depending on the procedure being done and the extent of the work. Typically, this is elective surgery and therefore not covered by insurance. But if it's done for dental or medical reasons, your provider may cover at least part of the cost.

ask the experts

What are the risks associated with chin surgery?

As with any surgery, bleeding and infection can occur. If an implant is inserted, the most common complication is **capsular contracture**, a hardening of the tissue around the implant that can result in an unnatural look. Also, the implant could be improperly positioned or shift over time. If an infection develops, the implant may have to be removed. While rare, you could have an allergic reaction to the implant material.

What is recovery like?

You'll experience swelling, bruising, numbness, or stiffness in the area—all of which can be relieved by applying cold compresses. Most of the swelling should subside in 2 to 4 weeks. If the incision is made inside your mouth, you'll be on a liquid diet for the first few days. You'll be able to return to work in a few days, but must avoid strenuous activity for at least 2 to 4 weeks. It will be 6 months to a year before the implant molds into the bone and looks its best. The results should be long lasting.

CAUTIONARY TALE

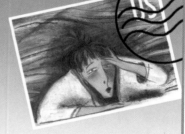

I needed a chin job, not a nose job

For years I had hated my nose. It was too big for my face. Everyone said so, even my mother! When I turned 30, I finally got the nerve up to see a plastic surgeon about fixing it. To my surprise, she said that my problem wasn't my nose, it was my chin. It was far too weak to handle the size and shape of my face. She suggested a chin implant and showed me via computer imaging what it could look like. I was amazed. I had the surgery done and sure enough, it really did transform my face. I now love my chin *and* nose. I wish I had seen a plastic surgeon much sooner—it would have done wonders for my self-esteem.

Phillipa S., Raritan, New Jersey

neck lifts

Trimming the fat from that turkey neck

Another harbinger of age is a fleshy, sagging neckline. Luckily, there are three procedures that can improve your appearance: **liposuction** and/or a **neck lift** to fix a fatty neck and sagging skin, and surgery to remove prominent bands or cords in the neck.

If you're younger than 40 and/or your skin has enough elasticity to snap back into place, a plastic surgeon can use liposuction (see page 138) to remove excess fat in the neck, thereby giving you a sharper, more defined angle in the jawline and neck. If you're on the other side of 40, in addition to liposuction, typically you'll need a neck lift, in which loose, sagging skin is removed via incisions made around each ear.

Another problem that some people are unhappy with is prominent bands in their neck. This is due to sagging neck muscles. To correct this problem, a plastic surgeon will perform a **submentalplasty** (also known as a **platysmaplasty**). With this procedure, your surgeon will remove the fat beneath the skin through a 1¹/₂-inch incision in the crease underneath the chin to access the platysma muscle in the neck. The muscle is then tightened either by lifting or cutting it to eliminate the pronounced cords. (Often, patients who undergo a neck lift have sagging in the jowls and cheeks, and so also have a facelift; see page 176.)

ask the experts

What can be done for my double chin?

Liposuction is often done along with removal of the **buccal fat pad** (the marble-sized fatty tissue that lies below each cheek). This combination of procedures creates a more sculpted, angular appearance for the face and neck overall.

What risks are associated with neck procedures?

Bleeding and infection can occur. With liposuction, too much or too little fat may be removed. With a neck lift, you may experience complications associated with the facelift, such as nerve injury and tissue loss. (For more on the facelift, see page 183.)

What is recovery like?

After liposuction, you'll typically wear a compression bandage around your neck for the first 24 hours and sometimes overnight for several days to aid in the retraction and shaping of the skin. If you've had a neck lift with a facelift, your doctor will likely put on a dressing to hold it in place for 24 hours to help reduce swelling. If you undergo liposuction, you may experience numbness and possibly a burning sensation in the area treated. After a combination facelift and neck lift, it takes 2 to 3 weeks to look near normal, 3 to 6 months until the swelling has largely subsided, and a year until your face and neck are fully healed. You won't be able to work or engage in vigorous activity for 2 weeks. You must limit your exposure to the sun for several months and use a strong sunblock afterward. The results should last 7 to 10 years—while fat removal lasts forever, the skin will sag again with age.

now what do I do?

Answers to common questions

I have an earring hole that is stretched out. Can I get that fixed?

Yes, you can. Your surgeon will cut away the skin around the hole to expose a fresh surface that can be knitted together. The hole is sewn up on the front and the back of the earlobe. This will then heal like a cut. This procedure, using local anesthesia, takes 20 to 30 minutes. After 2 weeks your ear can be repierced at a different site. The cost for closing up a hole in an earlobe is about $600 to $800.

Can I wear my glasses or contact lenses after facial surgery?

You may have to stop wearing glasses for the first few days or weeks following surgery of the nose or ears. If you must wear them, you will have to do so in a way that they will not rest on the bridge or ears, such as taping them to your forehead. You will not be able to wear contact lenses for a while after eyelid surgery.

Will I need to take extra precautions against sun exposure?

It's good advice to use sunscreen all the time, but it is especially important to use it after cosmetic surgery on the face and neck. In fact, most doctors require you to use a strong sunblock for several months after a procedure. (See page 30 for information about sunblock.) If you have work done around the eyes, you should also wear sunglasses that have 100% filters for UVA and UVB rays.

Should I tell my other healthcare providers that I've had cosmetic surgery on my face?

You should always tell your medical practitioners your complete medical history, including any type of surgery you've undergone, whether it was performed in a hospital or an outpatient facility, and whether you were given general or local anesthesia.

How can I build up my weak chin or jaw?

To enhance your chin you can get a synthetic implant, or you can undergo an **autogenous chin advancement**. For the latter, your surgeon makes an incision inside your mouth, cuts the lower jawbone and moves it forward, then wires the cut segment into its new position. For a stronger, more defined jaw, you can get a synthetic implant, which is placed right on the jawbone. Your surgeon makes an incision inside your mouth in the groove between the teeth and lower lip, separates the tissue from the bone to create a pocket for the implant, and inserts it. (For more on jaw restructuring, see page 110.)

now where do I go?!

CONTACTS	ADDITIONAL INFORMATION
American Academy of Facial Plastic and Reconstructive Surgery **www.aafprs.org** 800-332-FACE	**Welcome to Your Facelift** By Helen Bransford
	Lift: Wanting, Fearing, and Having a Face-lift By Joan Kron
American Society of Plastic Surgeons **www.plasticsurgery.org** 847-228-9900	**The Lowdown on Facelifts and Other Wrinkle Remedies** By Wendy Lewis
American Society for Aesthetic Plastic Surgery **www.surgery.org** 212-921-0500	Cosmetic Surgery News **www.cosmeticsurgery-news.com**
	Cosmetic Surgery & Skin Care News **www.cosmetic-surgery-news.com**

Chapter 10

The Facelift

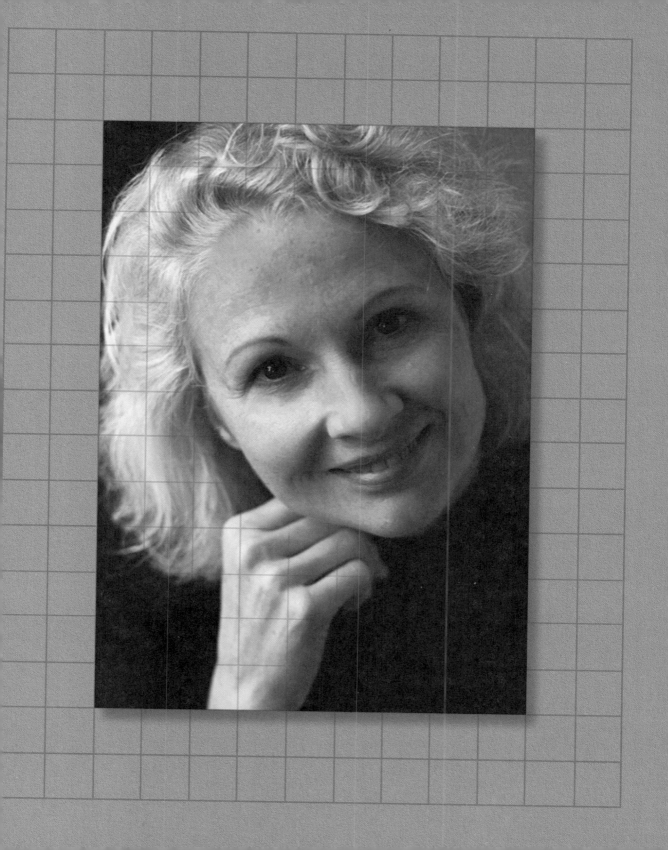

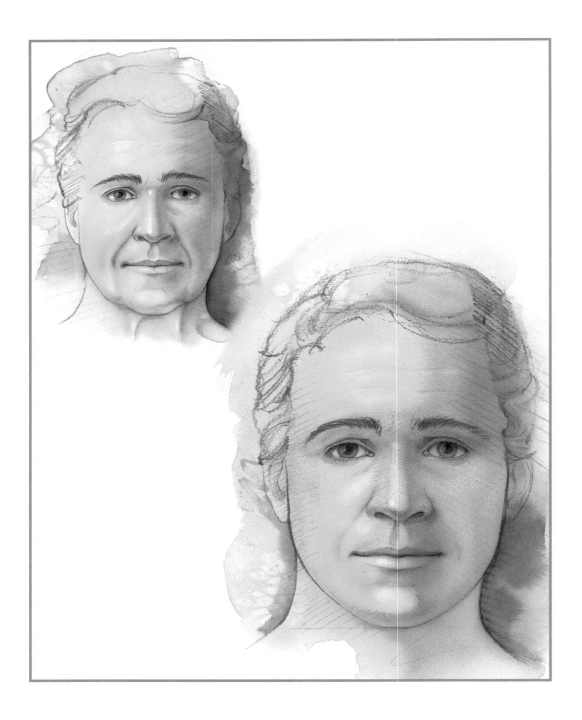

What exactly does a facelift do? It tightens the loose skin on your face and neck while addressing underlying muscle, tissue, and fat. The result is a fresher, firmer appearance. For many, the external results of a facelift can create an internal glow that will shine for years to come.

is a facelift right for you?

Attempting to turn back time

 h, the facelift. It is the crowning achievement of cosmetic surgery. In this 2- to 5-hour procedure the skin of the face is literally lifted off and repositioned. Why do this? Because age has a terrible of way of distorting our youthful looks. Time and gravity can alter our facial symmetry so that, for example, sagging jowls now make the face appear longer, and less pleasant.

To compound the problem, as we age our skin loses its tone and elasticity. The result? Wrinkles and creases as well as sagging skin. The "cure" for all these natural setbacks, including for the neck, is the facelift. It not only cuts away loose skin, it tightens it.

A facelift will not miraculously make you look years younger, but you can expect your face to look firmer and more refreshed. Once your surgeon has cut away loose skin and tightened sagging facial muscles, the results should last for 7 to 10 years. But even after a facelift, gravity and the aging process will continue to take their toll. So yes, you may want to repeat the lift. (See page 184 for information on the follow-up procedure.)

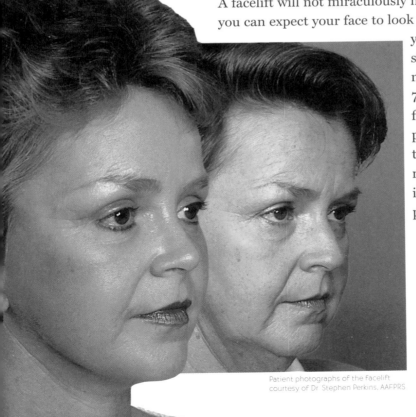

Patient photographs of the facelift
courtesy of Dr. Stephen Perkins, AAFPRS

ask the experts

How can I tell what I might look like after a facelift?

You can study your face in a mirror while gently pulling the skin with your fingers to mimic the effect (the real thing will look more natural). Or have your surgeon demonstrate this with his hands. Computer imaging is not very helpful for showing how you'll look after this type of procedure because there's no way to predict just how you'll heal.

What is the best age to have a facelift?

The best candidates are in their mid-40s to mid-50s, when the signs of aging begin to show in the face. Having the surgery done at this age, before things get too far gone, will yield a better outcome because there is still elasticity to the skin. Once skin has lost its elasticity it seems to sag faster, which is why first facelifts for people 70 and older aren't as successful.

the classic facelift

Put your best face forward

There are four main areas of the face where the sagging and bagging effects of aging are most apparent: those lines running from the corners of the nose to the mouth, the loose skin at the sides of the mouth, the jowls, and the loose skin under the chin (the neck). A facelift, or **rhytidectomy**, addresses all four problem areas at once. Unlike most other cosmetic operations, the facelift is surgery not to make structural changes (such as removing a bump in the nose), but to reduce the sags and bags in the face (and often the neck).

What is done during a facelift? Basically, an incision is made in the hairline from the temple down to the crease in front of the earlobe, around the back of the ear, and into the hair behind the ear. The skin is then lifted up off the underlying layers of fat and muscle and any excess fat is cut away or removed using liposuction (see page 138). The remaining fat is repositioned and underlying muscle tightened to restore the contour to your face. The skin is then pulled—or "lifted"—into its new position, toward the top or back of the head. Finally, excess skin is removed and the deep tissue and skin layers are stitched into place.

The surgery, using local or general anesthesia, can take anywhere from 2 to 5 hours to perform, depending on the extent of the work involved. A note for men: After a facelift you may need to shave behind your ears, where beard-growing skin will be repositioned.

ask the experts

What are the risks associated with this procedure?

There may be some bleeding in the first 24 hours after surgery, so you should stay close to your surgeon. If a large pool of blood develops under the skin (called a **hematoma**), your surgeon will have to drain it quickly to prevent tissue loss and scarring. A small hematoma, a common complication, is less a danger than a nuisance, as it will take many weeks to dissolve. Also, during the surgery, one or more of the nerves that control facial muscles may be injured; if they are bruised, the symptoms should subside in 3 to 12 months. But if a nerve is severed, the damage can be permanent. In addition, heavy scarring and infection can occur. There may also be tissue loss due to poor circulation in the skin. (Smokers run such a high risk for this that some surgeons refuse to operate on them.) If the skin is pulled too tight, you may end up with an uneven look or suffer hair loss if the hair **follicles** (roots) are destroyed at the hairline.

What happens after the surgery?

To minimize bruising and swelling, cold compresses and a bulky compression dressing are sometimes applied. For the first few days, you'll have to keep your head elevated when lying down. The day after surgery, your doctor will remove a suction drain inserted to collect any oozing. Because the sensory nerves around the ears are cut you'll experience numbness in that area. This should go away in 6 months to a year. You'll feel discomfort, but not terrible pain, for a few days, and your skin will feel tender, tight, and dry.

What is recovery like?

It takes 2 to 3 weeks to look nearly normal, 3 to 6 months for the swelling to subside, and a year until the face is fully healed. You cannot go to work or engage in vigorous activity for 2 weeks. After 3 weeks, you can resume all activities provided you don't feel any tension in the area. You should limit sun exposure for several months and then make a habit of using a strong sunblock.

FEES

Facelift

Surgeons' fees range from $4,000 to $14,000, depending on the extent of the work being done. If a facelift is performed along with other cosmetic surgery (on the eyelids or neck, for example), you should factor that cost into your total. Treatment for cosmetic reasons alone is not covered by insurance. However, if surgery is being done to correct a deformity or injury, you may be partially covered.

the second facelift

Follow-up procedures

It is quite common to redo a facelift. In fact, many people have two or three facial rejuvenation surgeries. The 7- to 10-year average lifespan of a facelift is a safe interval between procedures. If done properly, a second, or even third, facelift should not leave you with an excessively tight or artificial appearance. After three or four facelifts, however, the skin's elasticity will be so diminished that—no matter how well done the procedure is— another surgery may result in an overdone look.

A follow-up procedure does not require a full-scale repeat of the initial facelift—there is not as much tightening of the deeper layers and there will be less skin to remove. Only parts of the face that require a touch-up should be addressed in successive operations.

There is a trend toward removing less fat during both primary and successive facelifts and instead repositioning it. Unless you are very overweight, as you age your face begins to look more gaunt due to fat sagging down into your jowls. To recreate more youthful, fuller cheeks, your surgeon will move the fat back up over the cheekbones by undercutting the fat and lifting it, or by folding the fat back up to where it came from. A series of stitches is then made under the skin to keep the fat in position.

FEES

Follow-up

Surgeons' fees for a second or third facelift range from $3,000 to $12,000, depending on the extent of the work. As with a primary facelift, if you combine this procedure with related surgery (eyelids, for example), you will need to factor in that additional cost.

ask the experts

What might make me be a poor candidate for this type of surgery?

If you have very little sag, you may get only minimal benefits from the procedure, especially when you consider the cost and discomfort involved. At the other extreme, you may be disappointed if your sags and bags are so bad that you'll need a two-step facelift process within a year to achieve the desired results. If your skin is damaged from years of sun exposure, you will also have a less satisfactory outcome and will likely need some sort of skin resurfacing to help with the lines. (See pages 28 and 54 for more on skin treatments.) Other red-flag candidates include people who have diabetes, hypertension, or autoimmune diseases.

CAUTIONARY TALE

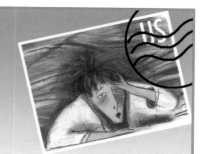

Not a facelift after all

I was growing steadily more unhappy with my appearance. I had just turned 52 and felt like I looked 72. My hair was thinning, and my wrinkles were all too apparent. It was time for a facelift. When I went to see a plastic surgeon he said the real problem wasn't my face—the wrinkles could be easily treated with a skin-resurfacing procedure. The real problem was with my receding hairline. It made my brow so prominent that my face was out of proportion. It prematurely aged me. He suggested a hair transplant. Well, I have undergone four hair transplant sessions and skin resurfacing. What an amazing improvement!

Red E., Waterville, Maine

mini-facelifts

The latest facial rejuvenation techniques

Techniques for traditional facelifts can vary, depending on whether your surgeon's focus is on repositioning the facial fat or muscle or—perhaps the real artistry to the facelift—how he or she redrapes the skin into its new position. However, the one common element is that the customary facelift involves an 8-inch incision that begins at the temple and moves along the crease around and behind the ear to the hair behind the ear.

A newer facelift technique is the **short trans-auricular rhytidectomy**, or short-scar facelift. Here, nearly half of the traditional incision has been eliminated. The surgeon makes small incisions around the earlobe, stopping before he reaches the hairline. Then he does the deep tissue work described earlier.

Other, newer techniques also call for much smaller incisions. In an **endoscopic lift**, for example, just a few small, strategically placed incisions are made in the hairline and an **endoscope** (an instrument with a tiny camera) is inserted into one of the openings to guide your surgeon.

In an **endoscopic lift**, your surgeon uses only a few, small incisions through which he cuts and recontours the tissue. This procedure is of benefit only in very particular instances.

These newer techniques had been performed primarily on relatively young patients who have very little loose skin, but now all age groups are possible candidates. The procedures are done in a hospital or outpatient facility, using local or general anesthesia. Note: These methods have not yet gained wider use because surgical advances of any kind take time for enough surgeons to have mastered them, and because some have limited applicability.

ask the experts

What are the major risks associated with this type of procedure?

Hematoma (a pooling of blood under the skin) is the most frequent complication. If it's serious, your surgeon will have to drain it quickly or it could cause tissue loss and extensive scarring. A small **hematoma** is less of a danger than a nuisance, as it will take many weeks to dissolve. Infection, abnormal skin healing, excessive scarring, and nerve injuries can also occur.

What is recovery like?

Because there is less cutting than with a traditional facelift, healing is more rapid. You will be able to return to work in 10 to 14 days. It will take about that long before you look near normal, 3 to 6 months until the swelling has largely subsided, and a year until the face is fully healed. You'll have to refrain from vigorous activity for 2 weeks. You can resume all activities after 3 weeks, provided you don't feel any tension in your face. You must limit your exposure to the sun for several months and always use a strong sunblock.

What can I expect from this surgery?

With innovations to the length and positioning of the incisions, both scarring and healing time are greatly reduced compared to that of the traditional facelift. Another bonus: Because incisions aren't made within the hairline (unlike traditional facelifts), there is little hair loss. As with the traditional facelift, the result from a mini-facelift should be evident for 7 to 10 years. But remember, gravity and aging will continue to take their toll after any type of facelift.

FEES

Mini-Facelift

Surgeons' fees range from $5,000 to $12,000. Treatment for cosmetic reasons alone is not covered by insurance. But if surgery is being done to correct a deformity or injury it may be partially covered. If you combine this procedure with related surgery (say, for the eyelids), you will need to factor in that cost as well.

now what do I do?

Answers to common questions

Will a facelift get rid of all my lines and wrinkles?

Many people incorrectly think a facelift, which minimizes sags and bags, can eliminate lines around the eyes, forehead, and other wrinkles. Such textural, not contour, changes can be addressed by procedures done in tandem with a facelift. (See page 28 for more on various facial treatments, and page 54 to get the skinny on how to improve lines and more with skin resurfacing.)

Will my face start sagging again the minute my facelift is done?

Post-operative swelling camouflages any sagging at first. You might begin to notice some sagging 3 to 4 months after surgery. Ideally, your facial skin should stay in place for several years before it begins to appear naturally loose, but not overly saggy. In disappointing facelifts, you'll see more sagging than you want in the first 6 to 12 months. Remember, though, having a facelift won't make you forever immune to the natural effects of aging. Your face will look firmer and more refreshed, but eventually it will begin to sag.

Will I need to take extra precautions against sun exposure?

After any cosmetic surgery on the face and neck, you must avoid prolonged sun exposure for several months. Cover up, use a strong sunblock, and wear a wide-brimmed hat. If you have work done around the eyes, you should also wear sunglasses that have 100% filters for UVA and UVB rays.

Should I tell my other healthcare providers that I've had a facelift?

You should always tell your medical practitioners your complete medical history, including any type of surgery you've undergone, whether it was performed in a hospital or an outpatient facility, and whether you were given general or local anesthesia.

What is a deeper facelift?

For certain individuals, more drastic procedures are emerging to tighten the face. Facelifts routinely involve lifting layers of skin, fat, muscle, and the **SMAS** (submusculoaponeurotic system), where the facial nerves reside beneath the layer of muscle. But in procedures like the **extended SMAS**, which calls for going deeper, and the **composite facelift**, which goes deeper still, there is a greater risk of permanent nerve damage and facial paralysis. Unless your surgeon can demonstrate that he has lots of experience, great success, and an ironclad reason for doing such profoundly deep surgery, choose a less risky facelift option.

Are there gender differences in doing a facelift and/or neck lift?

While the procedures for men and women are similar, men have factors that limit success, including wider, shorter necks and thicker skin. They bleed more during surgery. And a man's face is larger than a woman's, so the surgeon has a more extensive surface area to work on.

ⓝow where do I go?!

CONTACTS	ADDITIONAL INFORMATION
American Academy of Facial Plastic and Reconstructive Surgery **www.aafprs.org** 800-332-FACE	**Lift: Wanting, Fearing, and Having a Face-lift** By Joan Kron
American Society of Plastic Surgeons **www.plasticsurgery.org** 847-228-9900	**The Lowdown on Facelifts and Other Wrinkle Remedies** By Wendy Lewis
American Society for Aesthetic Plastic Surgery **www.surgery.org** 212-921-0500	Cosmetic Surgery News **www.cosmeticsurgery-news.com** Cosmetic Surgery & Skin Care News **www.cosmetic-surgery-news.com**

helpful resources

Certification for Doctors

American Board of Dermatology
www.abderm.org
313-874-1088

American Board of Medical Specialties
www.abms.org
866-ASK-ABMS (866-275-2267)

American Board of Ophthalmology
www.abop.org
610-664-1175

American Board of Oral
and Maxillofacial Surgery
www.aboms.org
312-642-0070

American Board of Otolaryngology
www.aboto.org
713-850-0399

American Board of Plastic Surgery
www.abplsurg.org
215-587-9322

American Dental Association
www.ada.org
312-440-2500

American Medical Association
www.ama-assn.org
312-464-5000

Accreditation for Surgery Facilities

American Association for Accreditation
of Ambulatory Surgery Facilities
www.aaaasf.org
888-545-5222

Accreditation Association
for Ambulatory Health Care
www.aaahc.org.
847-853-6060

Joint Commission on Accreditation
of Healthcare Organizations
www.jcaho.org (click on Quality Check)
630-792-5000

General Information (Referrals, procedures and more)

Academy of General Dentistry
www.agd.org
312-440-4300

American Academy of Dermatology
www.aad.org
888-462-DERM (888-462-3376)

American Academy of Facial Plastic
and Reconstructive Surgery
www.aafprs.org and
www.facial-plastic-surgery.org
800-332-FACE (800-332-3223)

American Academy of Micropigmentation
www.micropigmentation.org
800-441-2515

American Association of Orthodontists
www.braces.org
800-STRAIGHT (800-787-2444)

American Electrology Association
www.electrology.com
203-374-6667

American Hair Loss Council
www.ahlc.org
888-873-9719

American Society
for Aesthetic Plastic Surgery
www.surgery.org
888-272-7711

American Society for Dermatologic Surgery
www.asds-net.org
800-441-ASDS (800-441-2737)

American Society of Anesthesiologists
www.asahq.org
847-825-5586

American Society of Ophthalmic
Plastic & Reconstructive Surgery
www.asoprs.org
407-647-8839

American Society of Plastic Surgeons
(Plastic Surgery Information Service)
www.plasticsurgery.org
888-4-PLASTIC (888-475-2784)

Canadian Society
for Aesthetic Plastic Surgery
www.csaps.ca
905-831-7750

Canadian Society of Plastic Surgeons
www.plasticsurgery.ca

Cosmetic Surgery News
www.cosmeticsurgery-news.com

Cosmetic Surgery & Skin Care News
www.cosmetic-surgery-news.com

Food and Drug Administration
www.fda.gov

International Guild
of Professional Electrologists
www.igpe.org
800-830-3247

U.S. Pharmacopoeia
www.usp.org
301-881-0666

meet the experts

Samuel J. Beran

Samuel J. Beran, M.D., is a plastic surgeon in private practice in Westchester County, New York. He is known for his expertise in hair restoration. He has also authored and lectured internationally on such subjects as body contouring and facial rejuvenation. He received his medical degree from Albany Medical College, followed by a general surgery residency at Thomas Jefferson University Hospital in Philadelphia, Pennsylvania, and a plastic surgery residency at the University of Texas Southwestern at Dallas. Dr. Beran contributed to the Hair chapter.

cosmeticmd@earthlink.net

914-761-8667

Walter Erhardt Jr.

Walter Erhardt Jr., M.D., F.A.C.S., served as President of the American Society of Plastic Surgeons in 2001. He has a private practice in cosmetic and plastic surgery in Albany, Georgia. An authority on breast surgery, Dr. Erhardt has been a clinical investigator for breast implant studies. He received a medical degree from the University of Virginia School of Medicine and completed residency training in general surgery, and in plastic and reconstructive surgery, both at Vanderbilt University Hospital in Nashville, Tennessee. Dr. Erhardt contributed to the breast reconstruction section of the Breasts and Chests chapter.

erhardtmd@mindspring.com

229-432-9325

Lee A. Gibstein

Lee A. Gibstein, M.D., an expert on breast surgery, has a private practice in plastic surgery in Bay Harbor, Florida, and is an Assistant Clinical Professor of Surgery at the University of Miami School of Medicine. He received an M.D. with national honors from Hahnemann University School of Medicine and completed a general surgery residency at NYU Medical Center Tisch Hospital in Manhattan, and a plastic surgery residency at the Harvard hospitals in Boston. He also completed additional fellow-ship training in cosmetic and craniofacial surgery. Dr. Gibstein contributed to the breast lift, enlargement, and reduction sections of the Breasts and Chests chapter.
305-865-2802

Karyn Grossman

Karyn Grossman, M.D., is a dermatologist with a bicoastal practice in Santa Monica, California, and New York City. With a focus on cosmetic dermatology, Dr. Grossman has written and lectured extensively on chemical peels, facial scars, laser products, and fat injections. She earned her medical degree from Boston University, did her internship in Internal Medicine at the University of Michigan, and completed her residency and fellowship at Harvard University. Dr. Grossman contributed to the Skin Care Smarts, Laser Resurfacing, and Parts of the Face (lips section) chapters.
310-998-0040—California
212-879-9504—New York

Marc G. Lowenberg

Marc G. Lowenberg, D.D.S., is widely known as a "celebrity dentist." This New York City cosmetic dentist specializes in smile makeovers through the use of porcelain veneers, cosmetic bonding, bleaching, and gum lifts. Dr. Lowenberg graduated from New York University, College of Dentistry, and was granted a General Practice internship at Metropolitan Hospital in New York City. Dr. Lowenberg contributed to the Cosmetic Dentistry chapter (bleaching, contouring, bonding, and veneers sections).

www.lowenbergandlituchy.com

212-586-2890

Alan Matarasso

Alan Matarasso, M.D., F.A.C.S. is in private practice in Manhattan and is an Associate Clinical Professor of Plastic Surgery at the Albert Einstein College of Medicine. A premier facial and cosmetic surgeon, Dr. Matarasso has written and lectured extensively on the areas of the face, brow, eyelid, abdomen, and liposuction. He received his medical degree from the University of Miami School of Medicine in Florida, and trained in general and plastic surgery at the Albert Einstein College of Medicine–Montefiore Medical Center. Dr. Matarasso contributed to several sections of this book, including the Body Work (liposuction, excisional reduction procedures sections), Parts of the Face, and Facelift (mini-facelift section) chapters.

matarasso@aol.com

212-249-7500

Seth Matarasso

Seth Matarasso, M.D., is a dermatologist with a private practice in San Francisco, California, and is an Associate Clinical Professor of Dermatology at the University of California School of Medicine in San Francisco. He received his medical degree from the State University of New York at Buffalo School of Medicine and did his residency training at the Department of Dermatology at the Baylor College of Medicine, with a postgraduate fellow of Dermatologic Surgery and Mohs Chemosurgery at the University of California. Dr. Matarasso contributed to the Skin Care Smarts chapter, specifically on skin-care basics, injectables, peels, and dermabrasion.

slm_md@msn.com

415-362-2238

Jennifer Salzer

Jennifer Salzer, D.D.S., is an orthodontist in private practice in New York City. She is a graduate of Duke University and New York University College of Dentistry. She earned a degree in the specialty of orthodontics from NYU and is an expert on invisible tooth alignment. She lectures nationally on orthodontics and at training and certification seminars. Dr. Salzer contributed to the sections about braces and jaw restructuring in the Cosmetic Dentistry chapter.

www.drjennifersalzer.com

212-755-2333

David B. Sarwer

David B. Sarwer, Ph.D., is an Assistant Professor of Psychology in Psychiatry and Surgery at the University of Pennsylvania School of Medicine's Center for Human Appearance. He received his Ph.D. from Loyola University Chicago, and completed a post-doctoral fellowship in the psychology of appearance and body image at the University of Pennsylvania School of Medicine. Dr. Sarwer's research and clinical interests focus on body image and the psychological aspects of plastic surgery. Dr. Sarwer contributed information about psychological issues to the A New You chapter.

dsarwer@mail.med.upenn.edu
215-662-7589

Mark P. Solomon

Mark P. Solomon, M.D., F.A.C.S., has a private cosmetic and plastic surgery practice outside of Philadelphia, Pennsylvania. He is recognized for his innovative treatments, particularly on cosmetic surgery for men. Dr. Solomon received his medical degree from New York University School of Medicine and completed his plastic and reconstructive surgery residency at the Hospital of the University of Pennsylvania. He also completed a craniofacial and cosmetic surgery fellowship in Paris, France. Dr. Solomon contributed to the Body Work (augmentation of calves and buttock), and Breasts and Chests chapters (pec implants, male breast reduction sections).

www.marksolomonmd.com
610-667-7070

Geoffrey Tobias

Geoffrey Tobias, M.D., is in private practice in New York City and New Jersey. He is a clinical instructor at the Mount Sinai School of Medicine and Associate Chief of Head and Neck Surgery at Englewood Hospital in Englewood, New Jersey. Recognized for his development and refinement of pioneering techniques in rhinoplasty, Dr. Tobias travels throughout the country teaching these advanced techniques to other surgeons, and has recently been awarded top honors for his research in the field of nose reconstruction. He attended Tufts University Medical School and completed his residency at the Mount Sinai Hospital in New York City. Dr. Tobias contributed to the Nose chapter.

www.rhinoplasty.com

212-245-0202

Linton A. Whitaker

Linton A. Whitaker, M.D., Chief of Plastic Surgery at the University of Pennsylvania Medical Center, is regarded as a leader in aesthetic surgery of the face, born out of his pioneering work in craniofacial surgery. In 1988 Dr. Whitaker founded and became Director of the Center for Human Appearance at Penn (committed to the study and treatment of appearance-related conditions, both cosmetic and reconstructive). A graduate of the University of Texas and Tulane University Medical School, he did his internship at Montreal General Hospital in Quebec, his general surgical residency at Dartmouth Affiliated Hospital in Hanover, New Hampshire, and his plastic surgery residency at the Hospital of the University of Pennsylvania. Dr. Whitaker contributed to the Facelift chapter.

linton.whitaker@uphs.upenn.edu

215-662-2048

glossary

Ablative laser This laser removes the top layer of the skin, while nonablative lasers leave the top layer intact.

Alphahydroxy acid peels (AHA) These are stronger concentrations of glycolic, lactic, and fruit acids used to peel away the top damaged layer of skin on the face.

Areola The pigmented skin around the nipple.

Asymmetry Unevenness, typically for a paired part of the body, such as the breasts or ears.

Atrophic An area, such as a scar, that is depressed, or crater-like.

Augmentation rhinoplasty This procedure is done to build up the bridge of the nose or to reshape the tip to create a stronger profile.

Autogenous chin advancement A surgical procedure in which your lower jawbone is moved forward.

Blepharoplasty Cosmetic surgery of the eyelid area.

Body dysmorphic disorders (BDD) This is a clinically recognized mental disorder in which sufferers obsess about imagined defects in their appearance, often to such an extreme that it disrupts their daily lives.

Botox This substance, which is made from the toxin that causes botulism, is used cosmetically to paralyze the muscles that cause wrinkles in the upper third of the face.

Breast augmentation Cosmetic surgery to increase a woman's bustline by one or more cup sizes.

Brow lift Also known as a forehead lift, this surgical procedure addresses lines and sagging skin in the forehead area.

Buccal fat pad This fatty tissue, about the size of a large marble in an adult, lies just below the cheek area.

Buttock augmentation The cosmetic enlargement or enhancement of the buttocks.

Calf augmentation A surgical procedure in which an implant is inserted to add shape or definition to the calf.

Cannula A thin, hollow stainless steel rod used in liposuction to vacuum out the fat cells.

Capsular contracture A tightening of the scar tissue that the body may form around an implant.

Cellulite Lumpy, fatty skin with a dimpled appearance, usually in the thigh area.

Chin augmentation A surgical procedure in which the chin is enlarged.

Collagen Fibrous protein in the connective tissue that supports and strengthens the skin.

Composite resin A medical-grade plastic used in treatment of the teeth.

Dermabrasion A controlled abrading, or sanding down, of the top layers of facial skin to allow a firmer, fresher layer to emerge.

Dermal grafts Tissue taken from one part of your body and transferred to another.

Deviated septum A medical condition in which a blockage in the nasal passages can cause difficulty breathing, or recurring sinus infections.

DHT **Dihydrotestosterone** is the byproduct of the male hormone androgen, which contributes to hair loss.

Donor dominance Hair that grows in the horseshoe-shaped fringe going from ear to ear that is genetically programmed to always grow—except in extreme cases of balding.

Dyschromia Early brown spots and uneven skin tone that we first see on our faces as we age.

Elective procedures Treatment that you choose to have done to enhance your appearance and which are not medically necessary.

Electrolysis Treatment for hair removal in which a wire or probe is inserted into each hair follicle to deliver a low electric current that destroys each hair root.

Endermologie Temporary form of treatment for cellulite in which a high-tech machine applies a vacuum suction to the skin and underlying tissues to smooth the skin.

Epidermis The uppermost layer of skin.

Eversion A turning down of the eyelid.

Exfoliants Products that help clear away dry, flaky skin, and unclog skin pores, leaving the face feeling smoother and softer.

Fascia The dense layer of connective tissue between the muscle and the skin.

Gingivectomy The removal of gum tissue, also known as a gum lift.

Grafts Pieces of hair-bearing skin used in hair transplants.

Gynecomastia Male breast enlargement, a condition treated with breast reduction surgery.

Hematoma A collection or pooling of blood.

Hypertrophic An area, such as a scar, that is raised.

Intra-abdominal fat Also known as apple fat, which sits below the abdominal muscle and surrounds the organs.

Keloid A thick, raised scar that grows beyond the area of a wound.

Keratoses Scaly red spots on the face that first becomes apparent as our skin ages.

Laser hair removal Hair removal achieved through a beam of low energy that, when absorbed by the pigment in the hair follicle, permanently disables that follicle.

Laser resurfacing Also called a laser peel, this cosmetic treatment removes the top layer of damaged skin from the face.

Lasers A device that uses a beam of light energy to vaporize the surface of the skin at specific and controlled levels.

Lentigines or **liver spots** Dots and freckles that first become apparent as our skin ages.

Lift procedure A cutting away of excess skin.

Lip advancement A surgical procedure to lift the lip.

Lip augmentation A cosmetic procedure that enhances thin or droopy lips.

Liposuction The mechanical removal of localized fatty deposits that are resistant to diet and exercise.

Macromastia Very large, heavy breasts.

Malar augmentation Surgery to enhance the cheek.

Malocclusion A bite in which the teeth do not meet evenly.

Mastectomy The surgical removal of the breast.

Mastopexy A breast lift, which involves moving the nipple and areola (the pigmented skin around the nipple) back to a higher, more youthful position and, at the same time, reshaping the breast.

Matting Many fine blood vessels emerging in an area where larger blood vessels have been destroyed.

Melasma The most common and difficult to treat skin discoloration, which appears as brown marks on the face and typically occurs during pregnancy.

Mentoplasty The surgical enhancement, reduction or reshaping of the chin.

Microdermabrasion Use of a small wand filled with tiny particles to gently abrade, or scrape away, the damaged surface of the skin.

Micropigmentation The relatively permanent application, or tattooing, of makeup.

MRI Magnetic resonance imaging is a noninvasive diagnostic technique that produces computer images of the internal body.

Nasolabial folds Deep lines that start at the base of each nostril and go around the mouth and almost down to the chin.

Nipple/areolar complex The nipple and the pigmented ring of skin around it.

Nonablative laser This laser works by heating up the deeper layers of the skin while leaving the surface intact. The heat stimulates the formation of new collagen.

Occlusives These products (petroleum jelly, cocoa butter, mineral oil) trap the skin's moisture without being absorbed.

Otoplasty Surgery to reshape the cartilage and reposition, or reduce protruding ears.

Pectoralis implants Implants inserted into the muscle area of the chest wall.

Phenol peel A very strong peel that goes down to the reticular dermis, which is the level of skin just above the fat, to remove lines and wrinkles and other facial skin problems.

Trichloroacetic acid peel (TCA) This medium-depth peel is designed to remove the top layers of skin to allow a firmer, fresher layer to emerge.

Porcelain veneers Ceramic, tooth-colored material that is very durable and reflects light as natural enamel does.

Propecia A pill that will maintain your current hair count and generate some hair growth.

Ptosis A droopy forehead or brow.

Reconstructive surgery The repair of abnormalities caused by defects, disease, and trauma.

Rhinoplasty The aesthetic surgical reshaping of the nose.

Rhytidectomy A facelift.

Rogaine A topical medication that can prevent further hair loss and regrow hair.

Saline implants Breast implants that have a silicone shell filled with sterile salt water.

Scalp reduction surgery This hair replacement procedure involves replacing a bald spot with a part of the hair-bearing scalp.

Sclerotherapy A treatment for the removal of varicose or spider veins in which a chemical solution is injected into the unwanted veins to destroy them.

Septoplasty Surgery to correct a deviated septum.

Septorhinoplasty A procedure combining a septoplasty with a rhinoplasty to treat the nose for appearance and function.

Septum Cartilage that makes up the natural partition between the two air passages and extends from the nostrils to deep into the nasal cavity.

Seroma A collection or pooling of fluid under the skin.

Silicone implants Silicone is a polymer that can be produced in a variety of solid and semisolid forms for implantation in the breast, calf, and other areas of the body.

Slot deformity Transplanted hair that was growing on the sides of the head that is now in the center will continue to grow in its natural pattern, and could leave you with a slot, or groove, in the middle of your head.

SMAS Submusculoaponeurotic system, where the facial nerves reside beneath the layers of skin, fat, and muscle.

Soft-tissue augmentation The injection of filling material in the lower portion of the face to address fine lines. The most common material used is collagen.

Subcutaneous lift A surgical procedure that raises the brows without raising the hairline.

Spider veins Thin red veins in the legs.

Temporal lift This is essentially one third of a brow lift, and raises just lift the outer edges of the brow.

Traumatic rhinoplasty Surgery to treat a broken or damaged nose.

Tumescent lipoplasty A liposuction technique also known as super-wet lipoplasty, in which large volumes of saline solution mixed with a local anesthetic and adrenaline are injected into fat to make the cells easier to remove.

Ultrasound-assisted lipoplasty (UAL) A liposuction technique in which sound waves are used to break down and liquefy fat cells before they are suctioned out.

Varicose veins Large blue (and sometimes bulging) veins in the legs.

Veneers Custom-made, thin porcelain or composite laminates (resin shells) that are bonded to tooth enamel.

index

the author: up close

Jodie Green has been a top editorial executive at several leading publications and Web sites, covering everything from health to home, fitness to finance, and lifestyle to law. She wrote this book in response to her fellow baby boomers' complaints about receding hairlines, crow's feet, and sagging skin. Jodie splits her time between New York City and Philadelphia.

Barbara J. Morgan Publisher, Silver Lining Books

I want Cosmetic Surgery, Now What?! ™

Barb Chintz Editorial Director

Leonard Vigliarolo Design Director

Sharon Boone Editor

Ann Stewart Picture Research

Emily Seese Editorial Assistant

Della R. Mancuso Production Manager